IBADAN MEDICAL SPECIALISTS GROUP
2017

T0282319

Contemporary Issues in
Mental Health Care
in sub-Saharan Africa

editors
Olayinka Omigbodun
Femi Oyebode

series editor
Olufunso Adedeji

BookBuilders • Editions Africa

Published in Nigeria by
BookBuilders • Editions Africa
2 Awosika Avenue, Bodija, Ibadan
email: bookbuildersafrica@yahoo.com
mobile: 0805 662 9266; 0809 920 9106

Printed in Ibadan
Oluben Printers, Oke-Ado
mobile: 0805 522 0209

CONTENTS

contents cont'd ...

PREFACE

Seventy percent of the global burden of mental disorders is located in low and middle income countries (LMIC), including sub-Saharan Africa (SSA). However, in Africa, only 0.62% of the national health budget is allocated to mental health compared to a global median of 2.8% and 5% in Europe. The government is the source of funding in 62%of patients with severe mental disorder in the World Health Organization (WHO), Africa Region, the lowest of all the WHO regions, and lower compared to a global median of 79%. This is compounded by poor resources, with mental health outpatient facilities in WHO Africa Region being less that 10% of the global median. To address these problems, the WHO launched its Mental Health Action Gap Programme (mhGAP) in 2008, to scale-up mental health services in low and middle income countries (LMIC).

Culture plays significant and multiple roles in mental illness. It plays a role in the pathogenesis, elaboration and reaction to mental illnesses. Culture also influences the pathways to management, and in sub-Saharan Africa, about 40-70% of mentally ill patients first seek alternative treatment with spiritual and/or traditional healers. This usually leads to delay in seeking bio-medical help.

Preface

Cultural formulation is now incorporated in the *Diagnostic and Statistical Manual* (DSM) *of Mental Disorders* since the 4th edition with the main goal to assist clinicians in identifying cultural-contextual factors that affect therapeutic choices. The purpose of this book is to address some of the contemporary problems in mental health care in sub-Saharan Africa.

The book is directed to all policy makers in sub-Saharan Africa to aid decision making about the urgent need for sustainable and relevant mental health care strategies, and the important areas that need prioritisation. The book should be helpful to local and international researchers in formulating research questions relevant to the African continent and it will be of interest to medical practitioners and students in the region as adjunct to standard text books.

I am grateful to all the contributors for their time, effort and hard work in bringing this book to life. And I wish to express my sincere gratitude to my editorial colleagues, Professor Olayinka Omigbodun and Professor Femi Oyebode, for the invaluable expertise they brought to bear on the manuscript.

Olufunso Adebola Adedeji. MBBS, MD, FRCSEd.
Honorary Senior Clinical Lecturer,
School of Clinical and Experimental Medicine
University of Birmingham, United Kingdom
Series Editor, October 2017

CONTRIBUTORS

Jibril Abdulmalik, MBBS, MSc, MHPM, FWACP Senior Lecturer & Consultant Psychiatrist Department of Psychiatry, College of Medicine, University of Ibadan, Nigeria

Abiodun Abioye, MBBS, MRCPsych. MSc. Consultant Psychiatrist, Partnership in Care, London, United Kingdom

Olufemi Adebajo, MBBS, MRCPsych (UK). Cert Non-Clinical Psychopharmacology. Consultant Psychiatrist. BetsiCadwaladr University Health Board, Bangor, Wales, United Kingdom

Timothy Olaolu Adebowale, MBBS, D.Psych (Manchester), FWACP (Psych). Chief Consultant Psychiatrist and Director of Clinical Services, Neuropsychiatric Hospital, Aro, Abeokuta, Nigeria

Yetunde C Adeniyi, MBBS, FWACP, MSc. Child Psychiatrist, Child & Adolescent Mental Health, University College Hospital, Ibadan, Nigeria

Taiwo Adewunmi, MBBS. Consultant Psychiatrist, Tees, Esk & Wear Valley NHS Trust, Durham, United Kingdom

Babajide Adeyefa, MBBS, MWACP (Psych). Senior Registrar in Psychiatry, Department of Psychiatry, University College Hospital, Ibadan, Nigeria

Olatunji F. Aina, MBBS, FWACP. Professor of Psychiatry, College of Medicine, University of Lagos, Lagos, Nigeria. Editor-in-Chief, *Nigerian Journal of Psychiatry*

Olugbenga Akande, MBBS, MSc, MBA, MRCPsych. Consultant Psychiatrist and Medical Director John Munroe Group, Leek, Staffordshire, United Kingdom

Contributors

Akintunde Akinkunmi, MB, LLM, FRCPsych., FRCP, VR.
Psychiatrist. Chief Medical Officer (Reserves), HQ 2nd Medical Brigade, Queen Elizabeth Barracks, Strensall, York, United Kingdom

Cornelius Ani, MBBS, MSc, MRCP, MRCPsych, MD, (Res), Academic Unit of Child and Adolescent Psychiatry, Imperial College London, London, United Kingdom

Olusegun Baiyewu, MBBS, FMC(Psych), FWACP. Professor, Department of Psychiatry, University Hospital Ibadan, Ibadan, Nigeria

Tolulope Bella-Awusah, MBBS, MSc. CAMH, FWACP. Department of Child and Adolescent Psychiatry, University College Hospital, Ibadan, Nigeria

Oyewusi Gureje, MBBS, MSc. PhD. DSc. FRCPsych. Professor and Director of Institute of Neurosciences, University College Hospital, Ibadan, Nigeria

Ugo Ikwuka, PhD. Department of Psychology, University of Wolverhampton, Wolverhampton, United Kingdom.

Kwabena Kusi-Mensah, BSc, MBCHB, MSc. CAMH, MWACP. Department of Psychiatry, KomfoAnokye Teaching Hospital, Kumasi, Ghana

Olawale Lagundoye, MBBS, FRCPsych. Consultant in Addiction Psychiatry, Sheffield Treatment & Recovery Team, Fitzwilliam Centre, Sheffield, United Kingdom

Adegboyega Ogunwale, MBBS, PGD (Statistics), LLM, FWACP. Senior Consultant Psychiatrist, Forensic Unit, Neuropsyciatric Hospital, Aro, Abeokuta, Nigeria

Abel A. Ojagbemi, MBBS, PhD, FMCPsych, FWACP. Lecturer, Department of Psychiatry, University College Hospital, Ibadan, Nigeria

Contributors

Olayinka Omigbodun, MBBS, MPH, FWACP, FMCPsych. Professor and Head of Department of Psychiatry, and consultant in Child and Adolescent Psychiatry, University College Hospital, Ibadan, Nigeria. Director, Centre for Child & Adolescent Mental Health, University of Ibadan, Nigeria.

Femi Oyebode, MBBS, MD, PhD, FRCPsych. Professor and Head of Department of Psychiatry, University of Birmingham, United Kingdom

Helen Sasegbon, MBBS, MSc. FWACP. Psychiatrist, St Andrew's Healthcare, Northampton. United Kingdom.

Bode Williams, MBBS, MRCOG. Consultant Obstetrician, Liverpool Women's Hospital, Crown Street, Liverpool, United Kingdom

1
Emerging Mental Health Systems in sub-Saharan Africa

Jibril Abdulmalik and Oye Gureje
Department of Psychiatry
College of Medicine, University of Ibadan

Abstract

Globally, there is increasing realization that mental, neurological and substance use (MNS) disorders are significant contributors to the burden of disease and human suffering. The situation is worse in low- and middle-income countries (LMICs), especially in sub-Saharan Africa (SSA) where human and material resources are not readily available. The health systems in SSA are weak, with poorly implemented or non-existent mental health policies, outdated mental health legislation, and poor budgetary allocations. The situation is further compounded by widespread ignorance, stigma and discrimination, all of which act in concert to restrict access to care. The net effect of these factors is a huge treatment gap in most SSA countries.

However, there are glimmers of hope, with several positive developments indicating growing interest in improving mental health services in several countries. These include a number of collaborative cross-country hubs for mental health research among SSA countries, with or without external partners. There is also an increasing trend of mental health specialists returning from the diaspora to contribute to capacity building efforts and to the delivery of mental health services in their home countries.

Keywords sub-Saharan Africa; burden of disease; MNS disorders; mental health systems

1

Introduction

There has been a large improvement in the awareness of the need for improved services for mental, neurological and substance use (MNS) disorders as well as increased advocacy over the past two decades, with increasing emphasis on global mental health. These developments are a culmination of several steps which have had incremental add-on benefits for the cause of MNS disorders. These exciting developments have resulted in changes in sub-Saharan Africa (SSA), and this chapter will situate the emerging trends and changes that have occurred within the overall context of global mental health.

Burden of mental, neurological and substance use disorders

Mental, neurological and substance use (MNS) disorders are grouped together on account of shared similarities. Some of these similarities include symptoms due to dysfunction of the brain, social determinants exerting a significant influence on their onset and presentation, often running a chronic course and frequent association with stigma and discrimination (Patel, 2016).[1]

The contributions of MNS disorders to the global burden of disease (GBD) first came to light following the report of the first GBD study, which showed the significant burden attributable to MNS disorders (Murray & Lopez, 1996).[2] It is now established that MNS disorders contribute about 10.4% of the GBD, and, as a group, they constitute the leading cause of years lived with a disability (YLDs), accounting for about 28.5% of all YLDs (Whiteford *et al.*, 2015).[3] An appraisal of trends in the global burden of MNS disorders from 1990 to

2010 reveals an increase of 41% from 182 million disability adjusted life years (DALYs) to 258 million DALYs (Patel, et al, 2016).[1]

This global burden of MNS disorders imposes a heavy toll on low and middle income countries (LMICs), where the health systems are weak, funding and government priority for mental health are very low or non-existent, and stigma and supernatural ideas about the causation of mental illness are widespread. The World Health Organization (WHO) estimates that 70% of the global burden of mental disorders is located in LMICs, including sub-Saharan Africa (SSA); whereas, nearly 90% of the global mental health resources are domiciled in high income countries (WHO, 2005).[4] In SSA, the most disabling disorders for young people aged 10 – 44 years are MNS disorders (IHME, 2013).[5]

Treatment gap
Globally, the majority of people with MNS disorders do not receive treatment for their condition. This treatment gap is significantly higher in SSA and other LMICs, ranging from between 76.3% to 85.4% as compared with high-income countries (HIC) where the treatment gap ranges from 35.5% to 50.3% (Demytterae et al., 2004).[6] In Nigeria, only about one in five of those with serious mental illnesses in the preceding twelve months received any care at all (Gureje et al, 2006).[7] This situation is further exacerbated by the glaring inequalities in terms of available resources—human and material. This is starkly illustrated by the report that one HIC alone—the United States of America— has more psychiatrists than the two most populous countries of the world (China

and India), plus all the countries of SSA combined (Patel & Thornicroft, 2009).[8] This inequality in personnel is unlikely to stop any time soon, as there is a continuing trend of highly skilled health professionals, including mental health experts, who continue to migrate to HICs (Jenkins *et al.*, 2010).[9]

Increasing concern by researchers and the global mental health community has led to calls for the scaling up of mental health services and the reduction of the huge treatment gap particularly in LMICs (Prince et al., 2007; Saxena et al., 2007; Patel et al., 2007; Saraceno et al., 2007; and Whiteford et al., 2015).[10,11,12,13] Furthermore, there is compelling evidence that cost-effective interventions which can be implemented by non-specialists are readily available (Gureje et al, 2007a; Chisholm et al, 2008).[14,15] Thus, while acknowledging the reality of insufficient mental health personnel in these countries, current evidence supports the adoption of a task-sharing approach as a pragmatic and feasible means of successfully scaling up mental health care services (Thornicroft & Tansella, 2004; Abdulmalik & Thornicroft, 2016).[16,17]

The World Health Organization (WHO) has taken this call a step further, with the launching of the mental health action gap programme (mhGAP) in 2008, and the subsequent development of the mhGAP Intervention Guide (mhGAP-IG) manual. The mhGAP programme was launched to drive the process of scaling up mental health services and reducing the treatment gap, especially in LMICs. Consequently, the mhGAP-IG was developed as a practical manual for training non-specialist health workers to identify and offer basic interventions for priority mental health conditions in these countries, while mental health professionals provide training and supported supervision, as well as referral focal points for more complex cases (WHO, 2008).[18]

Health systems thinking and mental health

Increasingly, there is a recognition that efforts to scale up mental health services and reduce the treatment gap in LMICs and SSA, cannot achieve any meaningful success without strengthening the health systems of these countries (Gureje et al, 2015).[19] The WHO defines the health system as 'all activities whose primary purpose is to promote, restore or maintain health' (WHO, 2000).[20]

Thus, while the raison d'etre of the calls for scaling up mental health services has become self-evident, what is less obvious are the questions of what needs to be done, and perhaps even more importantly, how it should be done. These questions can only be answered through functional mental health systems. The challenge is greater in SSA where there is a neglect of issues relating to mental health (Minas, 2012; Jenkins et al, 2013; Abdulmalik et al, 2016).[21,22,23] Several barriers which continue to hinder the successful improvement of mental health systems in SSA and LMICs include insufficient personnel, poor funding, low government priority for mental health, health governance bottlenecks as well as communal perceptions which stigmatize and discriminate against persons with mental disorders (Saraceno et al, 2007; Abdulmalik et al, 2016).[13,23]

Current situational analysis of mental health in SSA

There is a paucity of information about the status of mental health services in most SSA countries but available data indicates a uniformly weak mental health system across the region with slight differences between countries. The following paragraphs present an overview of the current situation of mental health in SSA.

a). Prevalence of MNS disorders

Nigeria and South Africa are two SSA countries that participated in the WHO world mental health surveys. These surveys were nationally representative, community-based epidemiological surveys that were conducted across several countries in all the continents of the world with the aim of generating prevalence rates of MNS disorders among adults. The lifetime and 12 months' prevalence for any disorder were reported as 30.3% and 16.5% respectively for South Africa (Kessler et al, 2009; Jack et al, 2014)[24,25]; while the corresponding figures for Nigeria was 12% and 5.8% respectively (Gureje et al, 2006).[7] While the relatively lower figures for Nigeria may be partly due to under-reporting, it is probable that other SSA countries will also have prevalence figures within this range of reported prevalence (Esan et al, 2014).[26] Another large survey in Nigeria, this time of elderly persons aged 65 years and above, showed a lifetime and 12-month prevalence rates of major depressive disorder of 26% and 7%, respectively (Gureje et al, 2007b).[27]

b). Mental health policy and plans

The existence of a mental health policy and a plan is a demonstration of the government's commitment to a set of values, principles, objectives and areas of action towards addressing the mental health needs of their citizens. Several countries in SSA lack either a policy or a plan for mental health services. However, a few not only have policies, but are revising them to align with new realities, Both South Africa and Nigeria recently revised their policies in 2013 and new policies have been adopted in Ghana in 2012; Sierra Leone and Liberia in 2009; and Gambia in 2007 (Esan et al, 2014; Mugisha et al, 2017).[26,28] The major challenge of implementation however remains even in countries where policies exist (Mugisha et al, 2017; Petersen et al, 2017).[28,29]

c). Mental health legislation

The WHO Mental Health Atlas reports that only 55% of the countries in SSA have any mental health legislation (WHO, 2014).[30] However, even this figure is deceptive, when we consider that with the exception of Ghana and South Africa which recently revised their mental health legislation in line with global best practices, the majority of SSA countries operate obsolete mental health laws. For example, in Gambia and Nigeria, the mental health laws are several decades old. Even though Nigeria has a draft mental health bill, it has been under legislative consideration by the parliament for several years, attesting to the low political priority given to the process (Esan et al, 2014).[26] Currently, Uganda's parliament is also considering a bill to be enacted as the mental health legislation (Mugisha et al, 2017).[28]

d). Mental health financing

The WHO Mental Health Atlas estimates that LMICs including SSA countries have a median public mental health expenditure of $2 or less per capita (WHO, 2014).[30] South Africa and Nigeria spend about 3% - 5% of their health budgets on mental health—largely channelled towards tertiary facilities; whereas Uganda and Ethiopia spend about 0.9% of their health budgets on mental health (Petersen et al, 2017; Mugisha et al, 2017).[29,28] Gambia depends on external donor funding exclusively for mental health activities, while Ghana spends about 1.3% of their health budget on mental health (Esan et al, 2014).[26] Obviously, this level of funding is grossly inadequate and partly explains the parlous state of mental health services in these countries.

e). Human resources

The personnel available for providing services to people with MNS disorders is not only grossly inadequate but is further worsened by the increasing tide of migration of skilled health workers from SSA to HICs (Jenkins et al, 2010).[9] The WHO World Mental Health Atlas for example depicts the stark numbers of mental health professionals, with the number of psychiatrist per 100, 000 population as 0.05 for Ethiopia; 0.1 for Nigeria; 0.09 for Uganda; 0.28 for South Africa (WHO, 2014).[30] Liberia has one retired psychiatrist while Sierra Leone has two and The Gambia has none. The figures are slightly better for psychiatric nurses but are even worse for clinical psychologists. These shortages have their impact in reduced access to quality mental health care services to those in need.

f). Organization of services

The current emphasis is on tertiary facilities which provide mental health care services in the majority of the SSA countries. These function either as stand-alone neuropsychiatric facilities or as departments within tertiary teaching hospitals. The majority of these facilities are located in urban cities while the rural areas are neglected (Esan et al, 2014).[26] Efforts to ensure that mental health is incorporated into primary care and general medical services using the principle of task-shifting are currently being pursued in a number of the countries in SSA to bridge the ensuing treatment gap (Semrau et al, 2015; Gureje et al, 2015).[31,19]

g). Information Systems
Mental health systems cannot function or grow in a meaningful manner without information. Yet, nearly all SSA countries do not routinely capture mental health conditions within their health management information system (HMIS). For example, while very limited information about mental health is currently being captured within the routine HMIS systems in Ethiopia, Uganda, Ghana and South Africa, none is currently captured in Nigeria and other SSA countries (Upadhaya et al, 2016).[32] This dire situation needs to change as the imperative of recording and tracking data for MNS disorders within and across routine health care delivery platforms cannot be emphasized enough. Very little meaningful planning can take place without reliable data.

Emerging trends and the way forward
Significant and positive changes have occurred and continue to take place in SSA with respect to mental health research and efforts to scale up mental health services using the best available evidence. It is especially encouraging to note the

increasing trend of mental health professionals in the diaspora coming back home to provide technical support towards improving mental health systems, reviewing and updating mental health legislation, as well as participating in capacity building activities in their respective home countries. Another critical development which bodes well for the future of mental health services in SSA is the emergence of strong collaborative hubs of research between SSA countries, with a focus on mental health system strengthening, utilizing implementation science approaches. It is to be expected that these collaborative research efforts will generate sound strategies and innovative solutions for overcoming the current challenges bedevilling mental health services in SSA. Furthermore, they should coalesce and ultimately translate into an improvement in mental health services delivery and a reduction in the treatment gap. Some of the more notable research hubs are presented here:

i). The Mental Health and Poverty Project (MHaPP)

Mental health policy development and implementation in four African countries of South Africa, Uganda, Ghana and Zambia. The programme went on from 2005–2011 with situational analysis of the mental health situation in the countries, as well as an evaluation of the mental health policy status. These reviews were utilized to identify the challenges and barriers preventing the successful integration of mental health into primary care, including the mental health system difficulties. Furthermore, it utilized a mixed methods approach to generate innovative strategies for overcoming the country-specific challenges (Flisher et al, 2007).[33]

ii). Emerging mental health systems in low - and middle -

income countries (Emerald).

This is an European Union funded, multi-country project which aims to improve mental health outcomes in low- and middle-income countries (LMICs) by enhancing health system performance. It aims to achieve this objective by identifying key barriers within health systems, and offering health system solutions and recommendations for improving mental health services delivery (Semrau et al, 2015).[31] The participating LMIC countries are Ethiopia, India, Nepal, Nigeria, South Africa and Uganda. The European partner countries are Germany, Netherlands, Spain, Switzerland and the United Kingdom. The project is divided into discrete work packages, which cover capacity building activities (service users, researchers and policy makers); economic costing of MNS disorders including strategies for sustainable financing; successful integration into general medical services and the development and pilot testing of indicators for monitoring the mental health system performance. This comprehensive approach should generate a body of information that is practically useful for the participating SSA countries.

iii). Programme for Improving Mental Health Care (PRIME) This is a multi-country collaboration that involves Ethiopia, India, Nepal, South Africa and Uganda, which aims to generate evidence to support the successful implementation and scaling up of services for MNS disorders within primary and maternal health care contexts (Lund et al, 2012).[34]

iv). Mental Health Leadership and Advocacy Training Programme (mhLAP). This is a capacity building programme for policymakers, mental health professionals, media practitioners, and advocates for mental health– including service users and caregivers. It focuses on the five English speaking West Africa Countries of The Gambia, Ghana, Liberia, Nigeria, and Sierra Leone (Abdulmalik et al, 2014).[35] The programme is a partnership between the University of Ibadan and Australian Aid, through a grant managed by CBM Australia on behalf of the Australian Department of Foreign Affairs and Trade. The training holds annually in Ibadan, as a Residential 2 weeks intensive Course using a combination of didactic lectures as well as practical group projects delivered by a select faculty of multi-disciplinary International and Local Experts. Since inception in 2010, a total of 193 participants from 10 African countries have completed the training course. It is currently focusing on the human rights of persons with mental disorders in the participating countries.

v). The Africa Focus on Intervention Research for Mental health (AFFIRM)

This is a research and capacity development hub, established in the 6 countries of Ethiopia, Ghana, Malawi, South Africa, Uganda and Zimbabwe. It aims to investigate cost effective interventions for mental health disorders, and strategies for successful integration of mental health into primary care using a task-shifting approach. AFFIRM is led from the University of Cape Town, and funded by the National Institute of Mental Health (NIMH), USA (Lund et al, 2015).[36]

vi). Partnerships for Mental Health Development in Sub-Saharan Africa (PaM-D)

The long-term goal of PaM-D is to create an infrastructure to develop mental health research capacity in sub-Saharan Africa and to advance mental health science by conducting innovative public health-relevant mental health research in the region. The hub brings together, outstanding researchers and institutions from the five countries of Ghana, Kenya, and Liberia, Nigeria and South Africa in collaborative partnership to achieve major improvements in their health systems. It aims to achieve this objective, in partnership with government departments and non-governmental organizations by:

- Expanding services for persons suffering from psychosis
- Developing and implementing targeted programs of training and mentoring that build mental health research capacity on the continent
- Creating and supporting a critical mass of experts for innovative mental health research to address the region's mental health needs.

The Collaborative Shared Care to Improve Psychosis Outcome (COSIMPO) trial aims to design a collaborative shared care programme, implemented by providers of complementary/alternative medicine as well as conventional medicine; and test its feasibility and effectiveness in improving the outcomes of patients with psychosis (Pam-D, 2017).[37]

Conclusion
The mental health situation in SSA continues to have major challenges and difficulties but there are strong and emerging

trends that are systematically generating innovative strategies and solutions to help overcome and strengthen the mental health systems of the countries in the region. While the migration of skilled professionals from SSA to HICs continues, there is increasingly a reverse trend of returning back home by African specialists in the diaspora to contribute towards improving the system through a variety of activities.

References

1. Patel V, Chisholm D, Parikh R, Charlson FJ, Degenhardt L, Dua T, Ferrari AJ, Hyman S, Laxminarayan R, Levin C, Lund C, Medina Mora ME, Petersen I, Scott J, Shidhaye R, Vijayakumar L, Thornicroft G, Whiteford H; DCP MNS Author Group. (2016). Addressing the burden of mental, neurological, and substance use disorders: key messages from Disease Control Priorities, 3rd edition. Lancet. 16;387(10028):1672-85. doi: 10.1016/S0140-6736(15)00390-6.

2. Murray CJL, Lopez AD (1996). The global burden of disease: a comprehensive assessment of mortality and disability from diseases, injuries, and risk factors in 1990 and projected to 2020. Cambridge: Harvard School of Public Health.

3. Whiteford HA, Ferrari AJ, Degenhardt L, Feigin V, Vos T (2015) The Global Burden of Mental, Neurological and Substance Use Disorders: An Analysis from the Global Burden of Disease Study 2010. PLoS ONE 10(2): e0116820. doi:10.1371/journal.pone.0116820

4. WHO European Ministerial Conference on Mental Health. (2005). Mental health declaration for Europe: facing the challenges, building solutions. Helsinki, Finland: World Health Organization.

5. Institute for Health Metrics and Evaluation, Human Development Network, The World Bank. The global burden of disease: generating evidence, guiding policy-sub-Saharan Africa regional edition. Seattle, WA: IHME; 2013.

6. Demyttenaere K, Bruffaerts R, Posada-Villa J, Gasquet I, Kovess V, et al. (2004). Prevalence, severity, and unmet need for treatment of mental disorders in the World Health Organization World Mental Health Surveys. JAMA 291: 2581–2590.

7. Gureje O, Lasebikan VO, Kola L, Makanjuola VA (2006). Lifetime and 12-month prevalence of mental disorders in the Nigerian Survey of Mental Health and Well-Being. British Journal of Psychiatry 188, 465–471.

8. Patel V, Thornicroft G. (2009). Packages of Care for Mental, Neurological, and Substance Use Disorders in Low- and Middle-Income Countries. PLoS Med.6:e1000160. doi: 10.1371/journal.pmed.1000160.

9. Jenkins R, Kydd R, Mullen P, Thomson K, Sculley J, Kuper S, Carroll J, Gureje O, Hatcher S, Brownie S, Carroll C, Hollins S, Wong ML. (2010). International migration of doctors, and its impact on availability of psychiatrists in low and middle income countries. PLoS One. 5(2):e9049. doi: 10.1371/journal.pone.0009049.

10. Prince M, Patel V, Saxena S, et al. (2007). No health without mental health. Lancet. 370 (9590):859-77.

11. Saxena S, Thornicroft G, Knapp M, Whiteford H (2007). Resources for mental health: scarcity, inequity and inefficiency. Lancet. 370(9590):878-89.

12. Patel V, Araya R, Chatterjee S, Chisholm D, Cohen A, et al. (2007) Treatment and prevention of mental disorders in low-income and middle income countries. Lancet 370: 991–1005.

13. Saraceno B, van Ommeren M, Batniji R, Cohen A, Gureje O, Mahoney J, Sridhar D, Underhill C. (2007). Barriers to improvement of mental health services in low-income and middle-income countries. Lancet. 370:1164–1174. doi: 10.1016/S0140-6736(07)61263-X.

14. Gureje O, Chisholm D, Kola L, Lasebikan V, Saxena S. (2007a). Cost-effectiveness of an essential mental health intervention package in Nigeria. World Psychiatry. 6(1):42-8.

15. Chisholm D, Gureje O, Saldivia S, Villalón Calderón M, Wickremasinghe R, Mendis N, Ayuso-Mateos JL, Saxena S. (2008). Bull World Health Organ.86(7):542-51.

16. Thornicroft G, Tansella M. (2004). Components of a modern mental health service: a pragmatic balance of community and hospital care: overview of systematic evidence.Br J Psychiatry. 185:283–290. doi:10.1192/bjp.185.4.283.

17. Abdulmalik J, Thornicroft G. (2016). Community mental health: a brief, global perspective. Neurology, Psychiatry and Brain Research.

Vol. 22 (2): 101–104.

18. World Health Organization (2008). Mental Health Gap Action Programme (mhGAP): scaling up care for mental, neurological and substance abuse disorders. Geneva: World Health Organization.

19. Gureje O, Abdulmalik J, Kola L, Musa E, Yasamy MT, Adebayo K (2015). Integrating mental health into primary care in Nigeria: report of a demonstration project using the mental health gap action programme intervention guide. BMC Health Services Research 15, 242. doi: 10.1186/s12913-015-0911-3.

20. World Health Organization (2000). Health Systems: Improving Performance. World Health Organization: Geneva.

21. Minas H (2012). The Centre for International Mental Health approach to mental health system development. Harvard Review of Psychiatry 20, 37–46. doi: 10.3109/10673229.2012.649090.

22. Jenkins R, Othieno C, Okeyo S, Aruwa J, Kingora J, Jenkins B (2013). Health system challenges to integration of mental health delivery in primary care in Kenya- perspectives of primary care health workers. BMC Health Services Research 13, 368. doi: 10.1186/1472-6963-13-368

23. Abdulmalik, J, Kola, L. and Gureje, O. (2016). 'Mental health system governance in Nigeria: challenges, opportunities and strategies for improvement', Global Mental Health, 3. doi: 10.1017/gmh.2016.2.

24. Kessler R, Aguilar-Gaxiola S, Alonso J, Chatterji S, Lee S, Ormel J, et al. (2009). Special articles. The global burden of mental disorders: an update from the WHO World Mental Health (WMH) surveys. Epidemiol Psychiatr Sci. 18:23

25. Jack H, Wagner RG, Petersen I, et al. (2014). Closing the mental health treatment gap in South Africa: a review of costs and cost-effectiveness. Global Health Action. 7:10.3402/gha.v7.23431. http://doi.org/10.3402/gha.v7.23431

26. Esan, O, Abdulmalik, J, Eaton, J, Kola, L, Fadahunsi, W, Gureje, O. (2014). Mental Health Care in Anglophone West Africa. Psychiatric Services, 65: 1084 – 1087.

27. Gureje O, Kola L, Afolabi E. (2007b). Epidemiology of major depressive disorder in the Ibadan Study of Aging. Lancet 2007; 370:957-964

28. Mugisha J, Abdulmalik J, Hanlon C, Petersen I, Lund C, Upadhaya N, Ahuja S, Shidhaye R, Mntambo N, Alem A, Gureje O, Kigozi F. (2017).

Health systems context(s) for integrating mental health into primary healthcare in six Emerald countries: a situation analysis. International Journal of Mental Health Systems 11:7. doi: 10.1186/s13033-016-0114-2.

29. Petersen I, Marais D, Abdulmalik J, Ahuja S, Alem A, Chisholm D, Egbe C, Gureje O, Hanlon C, Lund C, Shidhaye R, Jordans M, Kigozi F, Mugisha J, Upadhaya N, Thornicroft G. (2017). Strengthening mental health system governance in six low- and middle-income countries in Africa and South Asia: challenges, needs and potential strategies. Health Policy Plan. 27. doi:10.1093/heapol/czx014

30. World Health Organization. (2014). World Mental Health Atlas. Geneva: World Health Organization.

31. Semrau M, Evans-Lacko S, Alem A, Ayuso-Mateos JL, Chisholm D, Gureje O, Hanlon C, Jordans M, Kigozi F, Lempp H, Lund C, Petersen I, Shidhaye R, Thornicroft G. (2015). Strengthening mental health systems in low- and middle-income countries: the Emerald programme. BMC Med. 10;13:79. doi: 10.1186/s12916-015-0309-4.

32. Upadhaya N, Jordans MJD, Abdulmalik J, Ahuja S, Alem A, Hanlon C, Kigozi F, Kizza D, Lund C, Semrau M, Shidhaye R, Thornicroft G, Komproe IH, Gureje O. (2016). Information systems for mental health in six low and middle income countries: cross country situation analysis. International Journal of Mental Health Systems. 10:60. DOI: 10.1186/s13033-016-0094-2

33. Flisher, A.J, Lund, C, Funk, M, Banda, M, Bhana, A, Doku, V, Drew, N, Kigozi, F, Knapp, M, Omar, M, Petersen, I, & Green A. (2007). Mental health policy development and implementation in four African countries. Journal of Health Psychology 12: 505-516.

34. Lund C, Tomlinson M, De Silva M, Fekadu A, Shidhaye R, Jordans M, Petersen I, Bhana A, Kigozi F, Prince M, Thornicroft G, Hanlon C, Kakuma R, McDaid D, Saxena S, Chisholm D, Raja S, Kippen-Wood S, Honikman S, Fairall L, Patel V. (2012). PRIME: A Programme to Reduce the Treatment Gap for Mental Disorders in Five Low- and Middle-Income Countries. PLoS Med. 9(12): e1001359. Doi: 10.1371/journal.pmed.1001359

35. Abdulmalik, J, Fadahunsi, W, Kola, L, Nwefoh, E, Minas, H, Eaton, J, Gureje, O. (2014): The Mental Health Leadership and Advocacy Program (mhLAP): a pioneering response to the neglect of mental

health in Anglophone West Africa. International Journal of Mental Health Systems 8:5. DOI: 10.1186/1752-4458-8-5

36. Lund C, Alem A, Schneider M, Hanlon C, Ahrens J, Bandawe C, Bass J, Bhana A, Burns J, Chibanda D, Cowan F, Davies T, Dewey M, Fekadu A, Freeman M, Honikman S, Joska J, Kagee A, Mayston R, Medhin G, Musisi S, Myer L, Ntulo T, Nyatsanza M, Ofori-Atta A, Petersen I, Phakathi S, Prince M, Shibre T, Stein DJ, Swartz L, Thornicroft G, Tomlinson M, Wissow L, Susser E. (2015). Generating evidence to narrow the treatment gap for mental disorders in sub-Saharan Africa: rationale, overview and methods of AFFIRM. Epidemiol Psychiatr Sci. 24(3): 233–240.

37. Partnerships for Mental Health Development in Sub-Saharan Africa (Pam-D). Available online from: https://www.nimh.nih.gov/about/organization/gmh/globalhubs/partnership-for-mental-health-development-in-sub-saharan-africa-pam-d.shtml. Retrieved 6th June 2017.

Summary

Learning points & objectives

- The burden of mental, neurological and substance use disorders is high globally, but is especially high in low and middle income countries – including sub-Saharan Africa (SSA).
- Mental health systems and the governance framework are very weak in SSA, with poorly implemented policies and outdated legislation.
- Insufficient resources (human and material) for mental health, and the poorly organized mental health services culminate in an unacceptably high treatment gap for MNS disorders.
- Several hubs of cross-country research collaborative programmes are increasingly coming to the fore in SSA with a focus on strengthening mental health systems, as well as integration into primary care.
- International migration out of SSA continues to occur, but there is a reverse trend of mental health specialists returning back to contribute towards improving mental health services in their home country.

Abstract

2

Pathways to Mental Health Care
in sub-Saharan Africa

Ugo Ikwuka and Femi Oyebode

Abstract

Mental health and culture are intertwined. Culture is a great determinant of mental well-being and state of psychopathology. The symptomatic expression of virtually all psychiatric disorders is influenced by culture. Again, culture can be a causative factor of psychopathology as obtained with Culture Bound Syndromes. Despite the importance of culture in mental health, its appropriate consideration in psychiatric diagnosis and formulation was not to be until few years ago when the concept of cultural formulation came into being.

Culture also plays vital roles in perceived aetiologies and effective treatment of psychopathologies in various cultures. In developing countries particularly, supernatural and preternatural factors are largely believed to be the causes of mental illness. Thus, the pathway to care/treatment in such environs is tortuous, with initial patronization of traditional healers before being taken to orthodox psychiatric facilities only after the traditional healers have failed.

Another important issue in cultural psychiatry is migration. With migration, many mental health professionals nowadays practice in cultures alien to their own. Thus, there is a recent emphasis on cultural competence, that is, acquisition of necessary skills to manage the mentally ill from different cultural backgrounds.

Keywords: Mental health; culture; culture and diagnosis; cultural competence; culture bound syndromes; migration and psychopathology.

Introduction

According to Parsons,[1] illness can be defined as

> . . . *a state of disturbance in the "normal" functioning of the total human individual, including both the state of the organism as a biological system and of his personal and social adjustments. It is thus partly biological and partly socially defined. Participation in the social system is always potentially relevant to the state of illness, to its aetiology and to the conditions of successful therapy.*

Thus, illness behaviour is a culturally and socially learned response, such that symptoms of any illness are differentially perceived, evaluated, and acted upon by people.[2] The factors that determine the response to illness include the visibility or perceptual salience of the signs and symptoms; the extent to which the symptoms are perceived as serious; the degree that the symptoms disrupt family and social activities; the frequency and persistence of symptoms; the tolerance threshold of the person experiencing the symptoms; available information and cultural assumptions of the person concerned; needs competing with illness responses; competing possible interpretation as to the causation of the symptoms; and, availability of treatment resources, physical proximity and the costs of treatment.[2] These factors are true for all illnesses. In this chapter we focus specifically on the potential response to symptoms of mental illness in sub-Saharan Africa.

It is well established that the pathways to mental health care are not random; while clinical factors such as symptom severity provide the impetus to the pathway as they do in physical illness, the decision to seek help and the selection of a help provider are structured by the convergence of personal, developmental, psychosocial, cultural, systemic and socio-economic factors.[3,4] From a cognitive theory framework,[5] three identifiable stages characterize the help-seeking pathway:

- defining the problem,
- deciding whether to seek help, and
- finding a source of support.

Research shows that pathways to mental health care largely follow three models reflecting the cultural and socio-economic characteristics of a group.

The biomedical model
The typical biomedical model characteristic of Western psychiatry is dominated by the biomedical explanation for mental illness with emphasis on the diagnosis of symptoms, which are treated primarily through medical interventions. Here, general practitioners (GPs) act as the gatekeepers to

psychiatric services. A deregulated form of this model where patients could see any health care professional of their choice with the possibility of having direct access to mental health professionals is also available in some parts of the world, such as Japan[6] and Eastern Europe.[7]

The 'free market' model

Alternative (traditional and spiritual) healers play important roles alongside biomedical professionals in the 'free market' model obtainable in sub-Saharan Africa. The consideration of a variety of treatment options in these contexts is mostly informed by multiple and sometimes conflicting beliefs being held as potential causes of illnesses.[8] This 'cognitive tolerance'[9] is reinforced by the holistic concept of human beings with the health and well-being of people attributable to immediate or distant social, spiritual and natural factors. [10,11]

Alternative institutional care in sub-Saharan Africa can be categorized into two types: syncretic religious (spiritual or faith) healers and traditional native doctors(herbalists). The two models often share a common recourse to the supernatural for both diagnosis and healing; faith healers to the Judeo-Christian God (or Allah for Muslims) and traditional healers mostly to a pantheon of gods or ancestors. Both often confirm the beliefs of patients and diagnoses are normally tailored to meet the expectations of the native clientele.[12,13] There is also a common tendency to mystify therapeutic procedures, which works to inspire awe in clients and dispose them more positively towards the therapeutic process. However, there are also significant peculiarities.

The spiritual pathway

Faith healers mostly belonged to the African Initiated Churches (AIC) though many have recently sprung up in the mainline Catholic and protestant churches. They adopt a Christian or an integration of Christian and traditional healing methods including religious rituals such as: prayers, fasting, prophesying, exorcism, deliverance sessions, use of sacramentals (holy water, holy oils, burning of incense etc.), offering of sacrifices, and the syncretic use of herbal medications and concoctions.[14,15]

The therapeutic process could involve: confinement, flogging, chaining, counselling, home visitation of patients to help them get rid of certain diabolical items which the healer claims had been used to bewitch the patient.

Some faith healers in the region also provide material support for the sufferers of serious mental illness who are also destitute. The faith healers place themselves at the meeting point between what they refer to as the backward and outdated traditional healers and the modern, scientifically-based Western medicine.[16]

The traditional pathway (1)

Traditional medicine is the sum total of the knowledge, skills and practices based on the theories, beliefs and experiences indigenous to different cultures, whether explicable or not, used in the maintenance of health as well as in the prevention, diagnosis, improvement or treatment of physical and mental illnesses.[17] Traditional healing practices could also involve medical and non-medical procedures including a series of complex rituals such as: divination, offering of supplications or sacrifices to appease the gods or ancestors (who could have inflicted the affliction), exorcism, use of charms and incantations (to ward off evil spirits), herbal medications and concoctions.[18]

The therapeutic procedure could also entail confinement, flogging, chaining and counselling. Traditional healers utter incantations to potentiate the medicine, which are regarded as possessing their own "life force" and not just the chemical activity of constituent substances.[19]

Diviners claim access to the supernatural realm, which enables them to unravel the cause of illness and misfortune. Hence, while laboratory services may be required to inform diagnosis and treatment in biomedical care, clients consult traditional healers for both causal explanations and the cure for their illness.

Traditional pathways (2): the social network
The social network is the network of potential consultants. It consists of multiple spheres of influence, each defined by its proximity to the individual; from the intimate and informal confines of the nuclear family through successively more select, distant, and authoritative laymen, until the professional is possibly reached.[4,3] The intervention of the social network is a significant aspect of traditional care in communitarian societies, which is what obtains in most of sub-Saharan Africa. The community in which one lives influences the conceptualization and interpretation of psychopathological symptoms, stereotypes regarding the effectiveness of given care pathways, coping mechanisms and the ultimate decision on which care giver to consult.[20]

The family forms the basic unit of the social network in these societies and is the customary starting point of the care pathway. Social networks can influence the help-seeking behaviour of people suffering from a mental disorder as a communication system by providing information and links, as a reference system by formulating normative expectations, and as a support system by providing care, reporting symptoms and helping patients cope with the psychosocial stressors, especially where the health care system is less developed.[21,22,23]

The decisive influence of these social networks was demonstrated in relatives initiating first treatment contacts in 91% of cases in southeastern Nigeria [24] and in 4 of 5 of cases in northern Nigeria.[11] Another study of northern Nigeria noted that sources of information about available mental health facilities mostly came from community members and neighbours (65%) ahead of the mass media (15%).[25]

While Western cultural values emphasize individualism, success, competition, and intellectualism, values that may inhibit westerners from turning to the informal network for help in fear that it may be interpreted as a sign of weakness,[26] family and primary group relations are central and most valued in communitarian cultures with emphasis on the collective over the individual. This enables mutual aid and reliance on informal help over professional mental health facilities, which from the perspective of the communitarian settings have the potential to isolate the patient.

Patterns of pathway use
A 'meta-analysis' of pathway studies in the region indicates

approximately an equal initial choice of biomedical (49.2%) and alternative (48.1%) mental health care pathways in sub-Saharan Africa.[27] However, regional differences could also be observed in the patterns of pathway choices. While studies from Nigeria (West Africa) and East Africa reported that more than half of patients initially took the alternative care pathways before arriving at biomedical psychiatric facilities, the reverse was the case in South Africa.

A study of southwestern Nigeria[28] reported that patients first consulted spiritual or traditional healers in over two-thirds (69%) of cases compared to 17.4% that consulted psychiatrists and 13.8% that consulted a GP. A study of eastern Nigeria[29] found that while 61.1% and 14.7% of the sample initially took the spiritual and traditional pathways respectively, only 9.2% took the biomedical pathway.

A study in southern Nigerian reported that more patients initially either consulted religious (48%) or traditional (20%) healers compared to the GP/psychiatrist (12%).[30] In northern Nigeria, over two-thirds (69%) of the patients visited religious healers, 28% consulted traditional healers, and 24% consulted GPs, while none of the patients first consulted a psychiatrist.[11]

A qualitative study in Uganda,[31] found that traditional healers were usually the first source of care people sought when faced with mental health problems, and frequently the only source of care sought. A study of an Ethiopian sample found that half of the patients sought traditional treatment from either a religious healer (30.2%) or a herbalist (20.1%) before they presented at the hospital, while approximately a third (35.2%) directly sought specialised psychiatric treatment.[32] However, Zimbabwe, southern Africa,[33] reported that biomedical care providers were the most commonly consulted at first instance.

Similarly, private sector GPs were mostly contacted (38.1%) in first instance in South Africa, followed by the police (23.8%), public sector general medical service (14.2%), mental health practitioner (9.5%), and traditional/religious healers (9.5%).[34]

Sixty per cent of respondents in a qualitative study of KwaZulu – Natal, South Africa, took the biomedical pathway as their first line of care while 40% took the alternative care pathways.[35]

As evident from the foregoing studies, research on the pathways to mental health care in sub-Saharan Africa dealt mostly with clinical samples that eventually presented at formal (biomedical) mental health care services where the customary pathway culminates. This creates a gap in knowledge since the pathways taken by many distressed persons do not lead to or end at such formal services. In response to this, Ikwuka[8] investigated the preferred pathways to mental health care by non-clinical respondents in southeastern Nigeria. While the study found mixed treatment preferences, as more than half of the respondents endorsed each of the three (traditional, spiritual, biomedical) treatment models, paradoxically, it found a significant preference for the biomedical (92.8%) compared to the spiritual (66.4%) and the traditional (54.4%) treatment pathways.

This corroborates another study of non-clinical samples that discovered that young Nigerian respondents favoured biomedical interventions and supportive environments as treatment models more than their British counterparts.[36] Arguably, these findings could suggest a paradigm shift from earlier prevalence of superstitious conceptualisations of mental illness in the region to an increasing scientific understanding possibly based on improved mental health literacy.

However, the findings could equally suggest a possible discrepancy between attitude (in non-clinical situations) and behaviour (in clinical situations). As symptom severity is a major determinant of help-seeking,[37] clinical samples would tend to be more pragmatic. When the mostly uninformed families are faced with an unforeseen onset of mental illness with some bizarre symptoms, fuelled by the deeply religious world view of the people, such 'strange' occurrences would naturally attract a supernatural attribution, that also discounts the effectiveness of biomedical psychiatry.

This explains why the majority of respondents in the earlier cited studies of clinical samples[29,24] who initially took the spiritual care pathway indicated that their reason for the choice was the belief that the illness was due to supernatural factors and their confidence in the spiritual care pathway. Crisis occurs when previous coping methods can no longer solve problems and in such situations people are more receptive to change.[38] As Angermeyer and colleagues[21] observed, if initial treatment experiences fail, the formal expert system is clearly favoured. This reflects the temporality of pathways and also explains why the clinical samples eventually turned up at the biomedical psychiatric facilities. Thus, help-seeking stages are not necessarily sequential or discrete, with individuals sometimes describing their getting help for a mental health problem as simply 'muddling through'.[3] However, pathways are travelled ultimately in the hope of attaining secure services, which may be reached in formal or informal settings.

Another variable capable of bringing discrepancy between attitude and behaviour in this context is the social desirability factor. Regardless of perceived efficacy of biomedical psychiatry, 'colonial mentality' is still evident in sub-Saharan Africa; the thinking that foreign (Western) products are superior to their local alternatives. Contempt for native systems has a structural link with the historical colonial demonization and the subsequent banning of African traditional beliefs and practices. Such a mindset is further reinforced in mental health care in the seeming 'imperiali-sation' of mental health as evident, for instance, in the Western creation of official categories of mental illnesses:

- Diagnostic and Statistical Manual of Mental Disorders (DSM)
- International Classification of Diseases (ICD), which have become worldwide standards.

Such biases also impose methodological limitations to pathway studies, whereby contacts with alternative services are usually underreported,[39] possibly because of the perception that informal contacts do not warrant equal status on the help-seeking pathway. Identifying with the 'superior' Western model would therefore be the more socially acceptable choice to make, especially by non-clinical respondents who are not under the pressure of symptom severity and who would therefore have the leisure of responding according to which behaviours are socially desirable.

Moving forward: Prospects of complementary care

Studies indicate increased recognition of the evidence base of biomedical care in the region. Clients in a South African study who expressed satisfaction with the treatment they received in district hospitals and mental health institutions based their contentment on significant reduction of symptoms they experienced following medication.[35] However, questions have been raised regarding the extent that biomedical psychiatric outcomes are culturally sensitive and inclusive.[40]

On the other hand, while traditional and faith healers may play an important role in addressing mental health needs by offering culturally responsive treatments,[41,42] these pathways are associated with long delays in reaching specialized services, hence a longer duration of untreated illness.[43,13] While the median time taken to reach specialist mental health services in Australia following the biomedical pathway was six months, with a significantly shorter time for patients with psychotic disorders,[44] the median delay between the onset of illness and the arrival at the psychiatric hospital in a study of an Ethiopian sample was 38 weeks.[45]

A study of a Nigerian sample[28] found that patients who first consulted GPs presented to an average of one care provider before presenting to mental health professionals, while those who consulted alternative services saw an average of six care providers before presenting to mental health professionals.

Delay is escalated by the lack of referral skills on the part of traditional and spiritual care providers, which may be fuelled by the conception of referral as admission of incompetence. Furthermore, though limited social networks predicted the restricted utilisation of mental health resources in a study,[46] research also hints at the irony of the inhibitory influence of tightly meshed social networks that can insulate individuals from linking up with biomedical health centres.[47, 4]

The foregoing demonstrates that no health care model is self-sufficient, nor are different models equally capable of rendering help quantitatively or qualitatively. It reinforces the call of the United Nations (UN) Permanent Forum on Indigenous Issues (2000) for a complementary approach to health care that envisages consultation with, referral to, or joint therapy with trained spiritual and traditional practitioners. Biomedical and alternative healers could help persons with mental illness by resolving different issues relating to the same illness.

Following Litwak's[48] formulation for instance, traditional kinship structures, resting on permanent relationships, can support long-term commitments to care; friendship ties, resting on free choice and affectivity, can support the provision of new information; based on geographical proximity, neighbours can deal with emergencies; while formal psychiatric institutions, resting on trained expertise and concentrated resources, can provide specialised segmented services.

Since mental health patients, especially those with psychosis, present early to traditional and faith healers in the region,[29] the constructive engagement with these providers could provide access to patients that is lacking for decisive early intervention. Dialogue with them needs to proceed with an openness that allows the possibility of cross-referral whereby the biomedical psychiatric model could, for instance, defer to the traditional model especially when conditions are scientifically inexplicable as could happen with culture-bound phenomena about which it has been observed that biomedical psychiatry has no satisfactory response.[49]

A complementary approach to care has worked effectively in a southern African (Lesotho) context[50] as well as in Europe.[51] In an imaginative programme in Hungary, pastors train alongside mental health professionals because of the observed link between people's mental health, religion and spirituality.[52] Pakistan equally exemplifies an innovative and comprehensive strategy specifically designed to take advantage of local opportunities to meet some of the challenges faced in developing countries. The strategy includes collaborating with traditional healers who have received some training, leading to increased identification and professional referral of individuals with mental disorders.[53]

The case for complementary care becomes all the more important in the face of the disturbing globalization of Western culture which presents just one version of human nature—one set of ideas about pain and suffering as being definitive. Adopting a strictly Western approach in these cultural contexts could, for instance, strip away the local beliefs that provide buffers and safe harbour in the face of crises. As Koenig[54] rightly observed, ignoring the beliefs of clients will cause psychiatry to miss an important psychological and social factor that may be either a powerful resource for healing or a major cause of pathology. While the pragmatics of a complementary approach in the region must be determined, training to promote improved cultural competency of local mental health professionals is a good starting point towards a bottom-up approach that recognises the importance of local conceptualisations of mental health difficulties for a more responsive service delivery.

Learning points & objectives
- Understand the concept of culture, and its inter-relationship with mental health.
- The role of culture in psychiatric diagnosis and management
- Understand the concepts of cultural formulation and cultural competence in current mental health practice
- Inter-relationship between migration and mental health
- The influence of culture on psychiatric stigma.

References
1. Parsons, T. (1951). *The Social System*. New York, The Free Press.
2. Mechanic, D. (1968). *Medical Sociology: a selective view*. New York, The Free Press.
3. Cauce AM, Domenech-Rodriguez M, Paradise M. *et al*. (2002). Cultural and contextual influences in mental health help seeking: a focus on ethnic minority youth. *Journal of Consulting and Clinical Psychology, 70(1)*, 44-55.
4. Rogler LH, Cortes DE. (1993). Help-seeking pathways: A unifying concept in mental health care. *American Journal of Psychiatry, 150*, 554-61.

5. Liang B, Goodman L, Tummala-Narra P, Weintraub S. (2005). A theoretical framework for understanding help-seeking processes among survivors of intimate partner violence. *American Journal of Community Psychology, 36,* 71-84.

6. Fujisawa D, Hashimoto N, Masamune-Koizumi Y. et al. (2008). Pathway to psychiatric care in Japan: a multicenter observational study. *International Journal of Mental Health Systems, 2,* 14.

7. Gater R, Jordanova V, Maric N. et al. (2005). Pathways to psychiatric care in Eastern Europe. *Br J Psychiatry, 186,* 529-35.

8. Ikwuka U. (2016). *Perceptions of mental illness in south-eastern Nigeria: causal beliefs, attitudes, help-seeking pathways and perceived barriers to help-seeking.* Unpublished Doctoral dissertation. United Kingdom: University of Wolverhampton.

9. MacLachlan M. (1997). *Culture and health.* Chichester, UK: Wiley

10. Westerlund D. (1989). Pluralism and change: A comparative and historical approach to African disease etiologies. In A. Jacobson-Widding & D. Westerlund (Eds.), *Culture, experience, and pluralism: Essays on African ideas of illness and healing* (pp. 177–218). Stockholm, Sweden: Almqvist & Wiksell International.

11. Aghukwa CN. (2012). Care seeking and beliefs about the cause of mental illness among Nigerian psychiatric patients and their families. *Psychiatric Services, 63*(6).

12. Edwards SP, Grobbelaar PW, Sibaya PT, Nene LM, Kunene ST, Magwaza AS. (1983). Traditional Zulu Theories of Illness in Psychiatric Patients. *The Journal of Social Psychology, 121,* 213-221.

13. Sorsdahl K, Stein DJ, Flisher AJ. (2013). Predicting referral practices of traditional healers of their patients with a mental illness: an application of the Theory of Planned Behaviour. *Afr J Psychiatry 16*(1),35–40.

14. Oyegbile, O. (2009). A Maddening Headache. *Tell Magazine, 22,* 47-50.

15. Lawani, AO (2008). The Nigerian society as a psychiatric patient. Paper presented at the Annual Scientific Conference and workshop of Nigerian Association of Clinical Psychologists. Benin City, Nigeria.

16. Freeman M, Motsei M. (1992). Planning health care in South Africa; is there a role for traditional healers? *Social Science & Medicine. 35*(11), 1183–1190.

17. World Health Organization (WHO) (2002). *Traditional Medicine Strategy 2002-2005.* Geneva: WHO.

18. Odejide AO, Oyewunmi LK, Ohaeri JU. (1989). Psychiatry in Africa: an overview. *The American Journal of Psychiatry,* 146, 708-716.

19. Nwokocha FI. (2010). *West African Immigrants in Northern California and their Attitudes toward Seeking Mental Health Services.* Unpublished MA Dissertation. California State University, Sacramento.

20. Sorketti EA, Zainal NZ, Habil MH. (2013). The treatment outcome of psychotic disorders by traditional healers in central Sudan. *International Journal of Social Psychiatry.* 59(4), 365-76.

21. Angermeyer MC, Matschinger H, Riedel-Heller SG. (2001). What to do about mental health disorder – help seeking recommendations of the lay public. *Acta Psychiatrica Scandinavica, 103,* 220-225.

22. Wong DFK. (2007). Crucial individuals in the help-seeking pathway of Chinese caregivers of relatives with early psychosis in Hong Kong. *Social Work, 52,* 127-135.

23. Bergner E, Leiner AS, Carter T, Franz L, Thompson NJ, Compton MT. (2008). The period of untreated psychosis before treatment initiation: a qualitative study of family members' perspectives. *Comprehensive Psychiatry 49,* 530–536.

24. Aniebue P, Ekwueme C. (2009). Health-seeking behaviour of mentally ill patients in Enugu, Nigeria. *South African Journal of Psychiatry, 15(1),* 19-22.

25. Abdulmalik JO, Sale S. (2012). Pathways to psychiatric care for children and adolescents at a tertiary facility in northern Nigeria. *Journal of Public Health in Africa, 3,* 15-17.

26. Tzahr-Rubin D. (2003). People's willingness to ask for help in time of trouble. *Haifa Forum for Social Work, 1,* 68-93.

27. Burns JK, Tomita A. (2015). Traditional and religious healers in the pathway to care for people with mental disorders in Africa: a systematic review and meta-analysis. *Soc Psychiatry Psychiatr Epidemiol. 50,* 867–877.

28. Adeosun II, Adegbohun AA, Adewumi TA, Jeje OO. (2013). The pathways to the first contact with mental health services among

patients with schizophrenia in Lagos, Nigeria. *Schizophrenia Research and Treatment.*Dec 31, 2013, 769161.

29. Odinka PC, Oche M, Ndukuba AC. et al. (2014). The aocio-demographic characteristics and patterns of help-seeking among patients with schizophrenia in southeast Nigeria. *Journal of Health Care for the Poor and Underserved, 25*(1), 180-191.

30. Jack-Ide IO, Makoro BP, Azibiri B. (2013). Pathways to mental health care services in the Niger Delta region of Nigeria. *J Res Nursing Mid 2*(2), 22–29.

31. Nsereko JR, Kizza D, Kigozi F. et al. (2011). Stakeholder's perceptions ofhelp-seeking behaviour among people with mental health problems in Uganda. *International Journal of Mental Health Systems 5*(5).

32. Girma E, Tesfaye M. (2011). Patterns of treatment seeking behavior for mental illness in Southwest Ethiopia: a hospital based study. *BMC Psychiatry, 11,* 138.

33. Patel V, Simunyu E, Gwanzura F. (1997). The pathways to primary mental health care in high-density suburbs in Harare, Zimbabwe. *Social Psychiatry and Psychiatric Epidemiology.*32(2), 97-103.

34. Temmingh HS, Oosthuizen PP. (2008). Pathways to care and treatment delays in first and multi episode psychosis. Findings from a developing country. *Soc Psychiatry Psychiatr Epidemiol 43(9),* 727–735

35. Mkize LP, Uys LR. (2004). Pathways to mental health care in KwaZulu-Natal. *Curationis 27*(3), 62-71.

36. Furnham A, Igboaka A. (2007). Young People's Recognition and Understanding of Schizophrenia: a Cross-Cultural Study of Young People from Britain and Nigeria. *International Journal of Social Psychiatry, 53*(5), 430-446.

37. Biddle L, Gunnel D, Sharp D. et al. (2004). Factors influencing help seeking in mentally distressed young adults: a cross-sectional survey. *British Journal of General Practice, 54(501),* 248-53.

38. Donnelly LP. (2005). Mental health beliefs and help seeking behavior of Korean American parents of adult children with schizophrenia. *The Journal of Multicultural Nursing & Health, 11,* 23-34.

39. Lincoln CV, McGorry P. (1995). Who cares? Pathways to psychiatric care for young people experiencing a first episode of psychosis. *Psychiatric Services, 46*, 1166-1171.

40. Vaillant GE. (2012). Positive mental health: Is there a cross-cultural definition? *World Psychiatry, 11:* 93–99.

41. Shibre T, Spangeus A, Henriksson L, Negash A, Jacobsson L. (2008). Traditional treatment of mental disorders in rural Ethiopia. *Ethiopian Med J 46(1)*, 87–91.

42. Abbo C. (2011). Profiles and outcome of traditional healing practices for severe mental illnesses in two districts of Eastern Uganda. *Glob Health Action, 4.*

43. Gureje O, Acha RA, Odejide OA. (1995). Pathways to psychiatric care in Ibadan. Nigeria. *Trop Geogr Med 47(3)*, 125–129.

44. Steel Z, Mcdonald R, Silove D, Bauman A, Sandford P, Herron J, Minas IH. (2006). Pathways to the first contact with specialist mental health care. *Australian and New Zealand Journal of Psychiatry.*40(4), 347-54.

45. Bekele YY, Flisher AJ, Alem A, Bahiretebeb Y. (2009). Pathways to psychiatric care in Ethiopia. *Psychological Medicine, 39*, 475-483.

46. Bonin JP, Fournier L, Blais R. (2007). Predictors of mental health service utilization by people using resources for homeless people in Canada. *Psychiatric Services, 58*, 936–941.

47. Birkel RC, Reppucci ND. (1983). Social networks, information-seeking, and the utilization of services. *Am J Community Psychol. 11(2)*, 185-205.

48. Litwak E. (1968). Technological innovation and theoretical functions of primary groups and bureaucratic structures. *Am J Sociology, 73*, 468-481.

49. Roe D, Swarbrick M. (2007). A recovery oriented approach to psychiatric medication: guidelines for nurses. *Journal of Psychosocial Nursing, 45(2)*:30-35.

50. Obioha EE, Molale MG. (2011). Functioning and Challenges of Primary Health Care (PHC) Program in Roma Valley, Lesotho. *Ethno Med, 5(2)*, 73-88.

51. Sevilla-Dedieu C, Kovess-Masféty V, Haro JM, Fernández A, Vilagut G, Alonso J. (2010). ESEMeD–Mental Health Disability: A European

Assessment in Year 2000 Investigators. Seeking help for mental health problems outside the conventional health care system: results from the European Study of the Epidemiology of Mental Disorders (ESEMeD). *The Canadian Journal of Psychiatry.* 55(9), 586-97.

52. Tomcsanyi T. (2000). Mental health promotion through the dialogue of different philosophies and professions: An interdisciplinary training in mental health. *Mental Health, Religion & Culture, 2,* 143–156.

53. Rahman A, Mubbashar MH, Gater R, Goldberg D. (1998). Randomised trial of impact of school mental-health programme in rural Rawalpindi, Pakistan. *Lance. 352,* 1022-25.

54. Koenig HG. (2008). Religion and mental health: What should psychiatrists do? *Psychiatrist 32,* 201–203.

3
Community Psychiatry in sub-Saharan Africa

Helen Sasegbon

Abstract

Mental health care is neglected in sub-Saharan Africa with less than 1% of health-care budgets devoted to it. Formerly, in Western Europe, persons with mental disorders were locked up in asylums, a model adopted in Africa as a result of colonization. However, community based mental health services have since become the preferred model of psychiatric care world-wide since they are more accessible and less likely to violate human rights. Community based mental health services include supported housing, psychiatric wards of general hospitals, local primary health care services, day centres and self-help groups.

Community based health services follow two models: the "Hive" with the hospital as the hub or the "Network" which is based on community resources. The "Hive" is the preferred model in Africa but is impeded by the scarcity of trained mental health professionals. The scarcity of trained mental health professionals impedes the development of community psychiatric services.

In southwestern Nigeria, the Aro Village system, based in Abeokuta was pioneered by Professor Thomas Adeoye Lambo who emphasized the importance of the treatment of persons with mental disorders conforming to cultural norms which in Nigeria involves the traditional healer and the involvement of the whole extended family.

Keywords: Community care; interdisciplinary teams; Aro Neuropsychiatric Hospital; MhGAP

Introduction

Sub-Saharan Africa (SSA) is the geographical area of the continent of Africa that lies south of the Sahara Desert, comprising 48 countries with a total population of 800 million in 2007.[1] The United Nations predicts a population of between 1.5 and 2 billion by 2050 for SSA and a population density of 80 per km^2 compared to 170 per km^2 for Western Europe.[1] Most countries in SSA are currently grappling with problems of communicable diseases, poverty, malnutrition and the lack of a safe water supply, which results in a poor standard of living and often life-threatening diseases. These health issues demand a huge outlay of material and human resources so that mental health issues have largely been relegated into the background.

Mental health systems governance has improved in Africa. In 2000, Gureje and Alem[2] stated that there was a need for a well-articulated mental health policy in most African countries where none existed. However, according to the World Health Organization's Mental Health Atlas, 71% of countries within the WHO African region have a standalone mental health policy, and 42% of these countries have updated their plans in the preceding five years.[3] However, only 14% of these countries have fully implemented these plans, and 41% have partially implemented them. Only 55% of WHO African region countries have a dedicated mental health legislation.[3]

In WHO, African region, an average of only 0.62% of the national health budget is allocated to mental health, compared to a global median of 2.82%, and 5% in Europe.[4] Government is the main source of funds for care, while treatment of severe mental health disorders in WHO African region at 0.62%, is the lowest when compared to the five other regions, and a global median of 79%. Out-of-pocket funding was the second most common source at 22%.[3]

In the past, Western countries treated persons with mental disorders in large psychiatric hospitals known as asylums, where they remained locked up for many years. However, partly as a result of the introduction of effective psychopharmacology, Western countries generally closed down or downsized these large psychiatric hospitals and advocated care in the community. This process of closing down the asylums is known as *deinstitutionalisation*, which is a process of replacing long-stay psychiatric hospitals with community mental health services for those diagnosed with a mental disorder or developmental disability.

The history of psychiatry in Africa is similar to the history of psychiatry in Europe. Lambo stated that the introduction of the European concept of mental disorder and its treatment into Africa came as part and parcel of the colonization process.[5] This was marked by the imposition of many alien institutions: political, administrative, and educational as well as the organization of health services, etc. After independence, various African countries introduced their own legal systems. Prisons were constructed and persons with mental disorders as well as criminals with mental disorders were incarcerated. In many cases, asylums were built for custodial purposes and there was no organized or scientific medical care for the patients.

Community-based care

However, in the world outside Africa, mental health care has moved in a different direction. World-wide, community-based mental health services have long been the preferred model of delivery of psychiatric care for a number of reasons. Chiefly, because they are more accessible and effective, since they lessen social exclusion. They are likely to have fewer possibilities for the neglect and violations of human rights than were often encountered in psychiatric hospitals. However, WHO also noted that in some countries the closing of psychiatric hospitals had not been accompanied by the development of community services, leaving a service vacuum with far too many not receiving any care at all.

Community care refers to a system of care in which the patient's community is the primary provider of care for people with mental disorders. The goal of community mental health often includes much more than simply providing outpatient psychiatric treatment. Community mental health services (CMHS) also known as community mental health teams (CMHT) support and manage people with mental disorders in a domiciliary setting instead of in a psychiatric hospital.

Thornicroft[6] provided a comprehensive definition of community mental health care as that which comprises the principles and practices needed to promote mental health for a local population by:

- Addressing population needs in ways that are accessible and acceptable

- Building on the goals and strengths of people who experience mental illnesses

- Promoting a wide network of support services and resources of adequate capacity

- Emphasizing services that are both evidence-based and recovery-oriented.

The spectrum of community health services tends to vary depending on the country in which the services are provided. Community services include supported housing with full or partial supervision (including halfway houses), psychiatric wards or units in general hospitals (including partial hospitalisation), local primary care medical services, day-care centres or club houses, and self-help groups for mental health, to help prevent and also to treat the problem.

In Western countries, a community-based mental health team is usually made up of psychiatrists, psychiatric nurses, psychologists, occupational therapists and social workers. In addition, there is collaboration between social services such as housing, various charities and other user organisations as well as telephone support lines. The role of the family is also vital.

Models of community care

The two broad conceptual models of community care that exist are the "hive system" and the "network system". In the "hive system", the hospital or "hive" is the centre of activities and there are various facilities such as day hospitals and clinics in the wider community. In contrast, the "network system" comprises a network of community resources and the hospital is only one of these.[7] The core of the service is a community-based multi-disciplinary team.

Tyrer[8] explained that the advantages of the hive system include an easier administrative system, a good range of professional expertise and many beds. Its disadvantages include poor accessibility for many patients, delay in referral, poor knowledge of community structures and the relative concentration of resources in the hospital.

They identified the advantages of community-based psychiatric services as easy accessibility, early contact with patients, sensitivity to the needs of the community and liaison with community services leading to continuity of care. The disadvantages of community-based psychiatric services include difficulties coordinating services, fragmentation of professional expertise and inability to provide a comprehensive range of services. While most mental health workers prefer the network system, it is the hive system that currently obtains in most of the countries in SSA.

Unfortunately, in SSA countries there are a number of factors that impede the development of community psychiatric services. One major factor is the scarcity of trained mental health professionals (table 1), and with such low figures, some African countries have no psychiatrist at all. However, there has been a 34% increase in the number of psychiatrists in Africa per 100, 000 population between 2011 and 2014 compared to a drop of 6% globally.[3] However, this increase in psychiatrists has been associated with an 8% drop in the number of nurses per 100,000 people over the same period.

Table 1. Mental health workforce by WHO region per 100,000 population.

	AFR	AMR	EMR	EUR	SEAR	WPR	World Median
Psychiatrists	0.1	1.1	0.9	7	0.4	0.9	0.9
Nurses	0.6	5.3	3.1	24.1	2.6	5.7	5.1
Psychologists	0	1.4	0.4	2.7	0.1	0.9	0.7
Social workers	0.1	0.6	0.3	1.7	0.1	1,5	0.4
Occupational therapists	0.1	0.3	0.2	2.1	0.1	0.9	0.2
Other mental health workers	1	5.9	1.4	11.8	1.5	6.2	3.7

AFR – African Region, AMR – Region of the Americas, EMR – East Mediterranean Region, EUR – European Region, SEAR – South-East Asia Region, WPR – Western Pacific Region.[3]

Table 2 below shows mental health facilities available in Africa (2011). Between 2011 and 2014, psychiatric beds in general hospitals, dropped by 15% each per 100,000.[3] WHO estimates suggest one outpatient facility per 3.31 million people in the African region compared to a global 0.17.[3]

Community resources

There is a paucity of governmental social services in most sub-Saharan countries and as a result, families, traditional healers and religious leaders are often involved in dealing with mental disorders. There is scope for more multi-sectoral collaboration and traditional healers may have a potential role in helping to provide community psychiatric care. However, this has to be carefully regulated.

Table 2. Facilities per 100,000 population by WHO region.

	AFR	AMR	EMR	EUR	SEAR	WPR	World Median
Mental Health Outpatient facilities	0.06	0.82	0.27	1.47	0.32	1.47	0.61
Day treatment facilities	0	0.02	0.004	0.310	0.003	0.230	0.047
Psychiatric beds in General Hospitals	0.7	1.3	0.5	10.5	0.7	0.5	1.4
Community residential facilities	0	0.010	0.012	0.211	0.005	0	0.008
Community residential facility beds	0	0.24	0.39	2.60	0.78	0	0.01

AFR – African Region, AMR – Region of the Americas, EMR –East Mediterranean Region, EUR – European Region, SEAR –South-East Asia Region, WPR –Western Pacific Region.[4]

Some of the early psychiatrists who practised in Africa, including Laubscher[9] and Carothers[10], stressed the need for extra-institutional provisions especially family care and emphasized the positive role of community resources as an important part of therapy. Cunyngham Brown recognized the importance of the family and stated that the asylum was not always the best form of treatment for the insane.[11]

An important example of one innovation that was made in order to deliver community mental health services in Nigeria was the Aro Village System which can be seen as the beginnings of community psychiatry in Nigeria.

The Aro Village System- an African innovation

The Aro Village System was developed in Abeokuta, a town in southwestern Nigeria, by Professor Thomas Adeoye Lambo (1932-2004), the doyen of Nigerian psychiatry. Lambo stated that the first village system for managing persons with mental disorders was instituted as a therapeutic strategy, utilizing the approaches of sociology, psychology, psychiatry and social anthropology and using the family and the community as the strategic focus.[5] Aro Village was operated as a training and research centre run by the Department of Psychiatry of the University of Ibadan.

Lambo began his experiment in 'village psychiatry' in 1954, in an attempt to draw on the resources available in village settings in Africa. Suitable patients from the psychiatric hospital in Aro were sent to live with their families in village locations close to the hospital. They were treated by members of staff from the hospital and continued to come to the hospital for consultation and treatment such as medication. Lambo stated that the African family and the community constitute an ideal strategic orientation for developing a therapeutic approach that is meaningful, economical and methodologically feasible.[12]

Very few innovations remain exactly the same as when they were started and the Aro Village System is no exception. Boroffka and Olatawura stated that the programme which was started as a "day hospital system"by Lambo had gone through various forms of expansion and modification.[13] Three of the original four villages that made up the system around Aro Hospital have dropped out and two others have been

added to maintain the original relationship with Aro
Hospital.

Adebowale[14] stated that the completion of the Aro
Hospital complex and wards and the subsequent developments of full inpatient care had gradually distanced the
community and even the relatives from patient care.[14] The
establishment of a new Directorate of Community Mental
Health Services in May 2006 by the Hospital Management
Board marked the first focussed effort to reestablish
community mental care following the *extinction* of the Aro
Village System of community care, to take the services of the
hospital into the community. The components of this service
include community outreach services, community residential
rehabilitation services, community partnership/liaison
services and community mental health day-care centre
services. This is discussed fully in chapter four.

There have been other innovations by Tigani El Mahi and
Taha Baasher who established working relationships with
Muslim leaders in Sudan, and others include, Asuni in Benin
(1979), Swift in Tanzania (1976), Margaret Field in Ghana and
Henri Collomb in Senegal (1976).

Community mental care and primary health care

Makanjuola[15] stated that those who have written about the
provision of services have agreed that there is a need to de-
emphasize institutional hospital care and move mental health
services in to the community, but opinions have differed as
to how this objective is to be achieved. WHO has proposed
the development of community mental health services

through the integration of mental health into the existing primary health care system and the mobilization of community resources.

The WHO definition of primary health care is essential health care made universally acceptable to individuals and families in the community by means suitable to them, through their full participation and at a cost that the community can afford.[16] According to Hollander[17] the primary health care approach is a system or process whereby health care is available at several levels.

The first level is the primary level in which there is contact between the patient and the health services. The secondary and tertiary levels are intermediate levels that provide more specialized health care facilities to which the patient may be referred from the primary level. The quaternary level includes the central referral hospitals and university medical schools. Patients may be referred up or down the chain.

Sub-Saharan countries differ widely in terms of their available current mental health services. It is important to note that African culture is not homogeneous and there is a diversity of ethnic groups and cultures in the eastern, western, central and southern areas of the continent with differences which must be taken into account.

According to Lambo,[18] psychiatric teaching and practice are based on the experience of Western societies, which may be inapplicable to the tropics. To be effective, psychological medicine must fit the relevant cultural pattern.

The services that do exist are also at various stages of development therefore the most practical and workable way of implementing community mental health services would be to incorporate them into the primary health care systems of the various countries, thus making best use of the existing systems. Ohaeri[19] speaking about developing a mental health policy and programme for Nigeria, advocated that in spite of their gross inadequacy, the existing mental health care facilities can be utilized as the basis of a stable foundation for meeting the ideals of health for all, if they can be integrated into the national primary health care scheme.

Alem[20] stated that there is a general agreement that mental health care services should be integrated into primary health care. A critical issue for the success of this model is perceived to be the provision of appropriate supervision and continuing education for primary healthcare workers. They also stressed the importance of collaboration between modern medicine and traditional healers. Boroffka[13] stated that the mental hospital in Africa, as in Europe and America, has forced itself into existence. It provided 'asylum' or shelter for the mentally ill in the past and he wonders about the type of place that will be offered in the future. He suggested that Aro Village, as with many other modern psychiatric institutions, combines elements of the traditional phase with those of the therapeutic phase and closes the circle, indicating, perhaps, future developments.

Lambo stated that traditional medicine, as applied to psychiatry in Africa, employs the concept of the 'family' or 'community doctor' in contradistinction to the concept of institutionalization.[5] In the treatment of psychological disorders, group therapy is the sine qua non and the whole extended family is often actively involved in forms of therapy such as singing, dancing, group confession, etc. The traditional healer's management of neurosis, psychosomatic disorders and personality problems remains unrivalled. This supremacy is recognized and accepted by Africans of all social classes, sub-cultures and affiliations.

In sub-Saharan countries there is an obvious need for the development of community psychiatric services which are geared towards the unique needs of specific socio-cultural groups. This is the only way that mental health care can become available to more mentally ill persons. The governments of sub-Saharan countries need to prioritize appropriate mental health care in their various countries as a matter of urgency in order to address the suffering of mentally ill persons. Extra- institutional community resources need to be developed further, utilizing indigenous resources when possible.

Lambo[21] summarized this succinctly when he stated that in planning and organizing mental health services, psychiatry in underdeveloped countries could profit from avoiding the mistakes already committed in advanced countries of the world. When Africa tries to abstract a lesson from European and American experience, she must make sure that it will apply to the contemporary African situation.

Developments
The WHO Mental Health Global Action Programme was endorsed by the 55th World Health Assembly in 2002 and the

next phase was the Mental Health Gap Action Programme (mhGAP).[22] This was WHO's action plan to scale up services for mental, neurological substance use (MNS) disorders especially for those with low and lower- middle incomes. It aimed to provide criteria to identify the countries with low and middle incomes which have the largest burdens of MNS disorders and the highest resource gaps, and to provide them with intensified support thus reflecting the continued commitment of WHO to closing this gap.

It identified several barriers to the development of mental health services, namely:

- The absence of mental health from the public health priority agenda with serious implications for financing mental health care.

- Mental health services centralized in and near big cities and in large institutions. These institutions frequently use a large proportion of scarce mental health resources, isolate people from family and community support systems and cost more than care in the community. They are also associated with undignified life conditions, violation of human rights, and stigmatization.

- The complexity of integrating mental health care effectively with primary health care services due to systems providing primary health care being overburdened. Limitations in human resources also contribute to this barrier, because only a few types of health professionals have been trained and super-vised in mental health care.

The mhGAP called for mental health to be integrated into primary health care and recommended that management and treatment of MNS disorders in primary care should enable the largest number of people to get easier and faster access to services. It stated that integration of mental health into primary care gave better care and cut wastage resulting from unnecessary investigations and from inappropriate and non-specific treatments.

WHO, Mental Health Action Plan 2013-2020[23] stated that in May 2012, the sixty-fifth World Health Assembly adopted a resolution on the global burden of mental disorders and the need for a comprehensive, coordinated response from health and social sectors at the country level. It requested that the director-general develop a comprehensive mental health action plan, in consultation with member states, covering services, policies, legislation, plans, strategies and pro-grammes. It stated that globally, annual spending on mental health was less than US $2 per person and less than US$0.25 per person in low-income countries, with 67% of these financial resources allocated to stand-alone mental hospitals, despite their association with poor health outcomes and human rights violations. The plan suggested that redirecting this funding towards community- based services, including the integration of mental health into general health care settings, would allow access to better and more cost-effective interventions for many more people.

The plan stated that the number of specialized and general health workers dealing with mental health in low- and middle-income countries was grossly insufficient and almost half the world's population lived in countries where, on average, there was one psychiatrist to serve 200,000 or more people. Other mental health providers who were trained in the use of psychosocial interventions were even scarcer. A much higher proportion of high-income countries than low-income countries reported having a policy, plan and legislation on mental health, with only 36% of people who lived in low income countries covered by mental health legislation compared with 92% in high-income countries.

One of the objectives of the Mental Health Action Plan was to shift the locus of care away from long-stay mental hospitals towards non-specialized health settings with increasing coverage of evidence-based interventions for priority conditions using a network of linked community-based mental health services, including short-stay in-patient, and out-patient care in general hospitals, primary care, comprehensive mental health centres, day-care centres, support for people with mental disorders living with their families, and supported housing.

This would be done by:

- Developing a phased and budgeted plan for closing long-stay psychiatric institutions and replacing them with support for discharged patients to live in the community with their families.
- Providing out-patient mental health services and an in-patient unit in all general hospitals.
- Building up community-based mental health services, including outreach services, home care and support, emergency care, community-based rehabilitation and supported housing.

- Establishing interdisciplinary community mental health teams to support people with mental disorders and also their families and care in the community.

- Supporting the establishment of community-based mental health services run by non-government organizations, faith-based organizations and other groups including self-help and family support groups.

Learning points & objectives

- Community care needs further development
- Culture plays important role is service set-up
- Centralisation of mental care is less patient friendly
- Integration of mental healthcare with primary care.

References

1. World Population Prospects-Population Division-United Nations. Esa.un.org 2015-07-29. Retrieved 2017-07-03.

2. Gureje O, Alem A. (2000). Mental health policy development in Africa. *Bulletin of the World Health Organization*.78(4):475-82.

3. World Health Organisation. (2014). Mental Health Atlas, Geneva: WHO

4. World Health Organisation. (2011). Mental Health Atlas, Geneva: WHO

5. Lambo TA. (1975). Mid and West Africa in history of psychiatry. 579-599.

6. Thornicroft G, Deb T, Henderson C. (2016). Community mental health care worldwide: current status and further developments. *World Psychiatry*, 15: 276-286

7. Peet M. (1986). Network community mental healthcare in North-West Derbyshire. *Bull. Roy. Coll. Psychiat*.10:262.

8. Tyrer P. (1985). The hive system: a model for a psychiatric service. *British Journal of Psychiatry*. 571-57

9. Laubscher BJF. (1937). *Sex, custom, and psychopathology: a study of South African pagan natives*. London: Routledge

10. Carothers JC. (1953). *The African may in health and disease: a study in ethnopsychiatry*. Geneva: World Health Organization.

11. Cunyngham Brown R. (1938). *Report III on the care and treatment of lunatics in the British West African colonies; Nigeria*. UK: Garden City Press.

12. Lambo TA. (1966). The Nigerian Village Program. In David HP. (ed.) *International trends in mental health*. New York: McGraw-Hill.

13. Boroffka A, Olatawura MO. (1977). Community psychiatry in Nigeria: the current status. *International Journal of Social Psychiatry*

14. Adebowale, TO. (2009). Paper presented at the World Psychiatric Association International Congress on Treatments in Psychiatry; An update April 1-4 2009, Florence Italy.

15. Makanjuola JDA, Odejide AO, Erinosho OA. (1990). The integration of mental health into primary health care in Nigeria. Department of Planning, Research and Statistics. Federal Ministry of Health, Lagos.

16. World Health Organization (1978). Mental disorders: glossary and guide to their classification in accordance with the 9th revision of the International Classification of Diseases. Geneva: WHO

17. Hollander D. (1998). *Developing mental health services: a manual*. London: Concern Publications.

18. Lambo TA. (1965). Psychiatry in the tropics. *Lancet* 286,7422:119-1121.

19. Ohaeri, JU. Integrating mental health care into the primary health care system in Nigeria. Paper presented at the seminar meeting of the committee to develop mental health policy and programme for Nigeria, Lagos, 26th June-1st August, 1989.

20. Alem A, Jacobsson L, Hanlon C. (2008). Community-based mental health care in Africa: mental health workers' views. *World Psychiatry*. 7(1):54-7.

21. Lambo TA. (1960). Further neuropsychiatric observations in Nigeria. *British Medical Journal*. 1696-1704.

22. World Health Organization (2008). Mental Health Gap Action Programme (mhGAP): scaling up care for mental, neurological and substance abuse disorders. Geneva: WHO

23. WHO 2013. Mental health action plan 2013-2020.

Other selected readings

Atalay A, Jacobson L, Hanlon C. (2008). Community-based mental health care in Africa: mental health worker's views. *World Psychiatry*. 7(1): 54-57.

Bitta M, Kariuki SM, Chengo E, Newton CRJC. An overview of mental health care system in Kilifi, Kenya: results from an initial assessment using the World Health Organization's assessment Instrument for Mental Health Systems. *Int J Ment Health Syst*, 11:28.

Forster EB. (2012). A historical survey of psychiatric practice in Ghana, *Ghana Med J*; 46 (3): 158-162.

Freeman HL, Fryers T, Henderson J. (1985). Mental health services in Europe; 10 years on. WHO Regional Office for Europe.

From Asylum to Hospital, Psychiatric Hospital Yaba 1907-1987, A publication in commemoration of the 80th Anniversary of the Hospital.

Gureje O. (2003). Revisiting the national mental health policy for Nigeria. *Archives of Ibadan Medicine*, 4.1: 2-4.

Hanlon C, Wondimagegn D, Alem A. (2010). Lessons learned in developing community mental health care in Africa. *World Psychiatry*, 9: 185-189.

Hollander D. Developing mental health systems policies and strategies for the development of mental health systems: an introductory overview.

Kigozi F, Ssebunnya J, Kizza D, Cooper S, Ndyanabangi S. An overview of Uganda's mental health care system; results from an assessment using the world health organization's assessment instrument for mental health systems (WHO-AIMS).

Marangu, E, Sands, N, Rolley, J, Ndetei, D, and Mansouri, F. Mental Healthcare in Kenya: Exploring optimal conditions for capacity building. *Afr JPrm Health Care Fam Med*. 2014;6(1).

Mental Health Action Plan 2013-2020, World Health Organization

MhGAP Mental Health Gap Action Programme, Scaling up care for mental, neurological, and substance use disorders, World Health Organization

Njenga, F. Focus on Psychiatry in East Africa, *The British Journal of Psychiatry* Oct 2002, 181 (4) 354-359

Roberts, M, Asare, J, Mogan, C, Adjase, E.T., Osei, A. June 2013 The mental health system in Ghana, fullrReport

Roberts, M, Mogan, C, Asare, J. An overview of Ghana's mental health system: results from an assessment using the World Health Organization's Assessment Instrument for Mental Health Systems (WHO-AIMS)

4

Community Mental Health Service Delivery at the Neuropsychiatric Hospital Aro Abeokuta

Timothy Olaolu Adebowale

Abstract

The Neuropsychiatric Hospital, Aro, Abeokuta, Ogun State was established in 1944 initially as an asylum at Lantoro. The purpose built hospital, located at Aro, started receiving patients about a decade later, in 1954. Aro Neuropsychiatric Hospital has enjoyed a rich historical legacy as the first purpose built psychiatric hospital in Nigeria. The hospital came into global limelight as a result of the novel Aro village system of care.

Aro Neuropsychiatric Hospital initiated and has continued to support the implementation of a state-wide programme for the integration of mental health care (MHC) into primary health care (PHC) in all local government areas (LGAs) of Ogun State in 2011. This process of integration was recognized as a landmark achievement for mental health service delivery in Nigeria, and the hospital received the National Health Care Excellence Award for Primary Health Care Service Innovation in 2015. Aro Neuropsychiatric Hospital management has introduced several strategies aimed at reducing the stigma associated with its use in last decade. This has been carried out through the deliberate 'opening up' and the establishment of a general medical practice clinic run by a consultant family physician, and medical officers.

Keywords: Aro Neuropsychiatric Hospital; integrated health care programmes; de-stigmatization

Changing service delivery at Aro Neuropsychiatric Hospital

Mental health service delivery at the Neuropsychiatric Hospital, Aro has undergone tremendous development from its inception in the 1950s with the introduction of evidence-based care of persons with mental disorders in the 1980s. Patronage of the Aro Village system of care during this period reduced drastically due to factors such as urbanization of the villages around the hospital, preference for full in-patient care for patients with difficult to manage symptoms and the need for relatives to return to their place of work, while the patient continues to receive care as an in-patient.

The beginning of the residency training programme in the 1980s and efforts towards the development of sub-specialisations in service delivery marked a period for mental health service delivery in Aro. All these advancements, however, further reinforced the institutionalized and stigmatised the perception of mental health service delivery in the eye of the public.

The new millennium marked a turning point in the history of that hospital with the concerted effort at winning the age long battle with the negative public perception of the institution as a psychiatric hospital. Two pronged strategies of 'opening up' and 'going out' were adopted.

The de-stigmatising strategies ('opening up')

One of the de-stigmatising/opening up strategies of the Aro Neuropsychiatric Hospital Management was the establishment of a community National Health Insurance Scheme (NHIS) clinic in 2005, with the appointment of consultant family physicians within the hospital premises. The clinic currently provides primary and secondary general medical services to members of the public who live in the communities surrounding the hospital, thereby fast changing the status of Aro as a psychiatric hospital. The climax of this de-stigmatisation step was achieved in 2012, when the clinic took the first delivery of a baby, of a member the community. Many deliveries have followed since.

Some of the other deliberate 'opening up' strategies of the hospital management since the early 2000s include the establishment of a Physiotherapy Department and a gymnasium; the opening up of a hospital conference hall and a cafeteria for use by community members for social events and activities; the conversion of some residential quarters into guest houses for hospital guests and members of the community. The hospital grounds and football field were also opened up for sporting activities by members of the community.

Community mental health programme ('going out')

Community activities (going out) of the hospital commenced officially with the establishment of the Directorate of Community Mental Health Services in 2005. The directorate has several educational and enlightenment programmes.

Intensive mental health education and enlightenment campaigns to special community groups such as secondary school students and artisans were commenced in 2007. The hospital secured and paid for a slot on Nigerian Television Authority (NTA), Abeokuta every Tuesday from 7.30p.m. – 8.00p.m. for a programme titled: 'Mental Health'. Various topics and issues on mental health were discussed between June 2007 and July 2008. The programme included a live phone-in session,. Community mental health enlightenment drama displays were also performed at community halls in Abeokuta and these attracted large numbers of members of the community.

Consultation and outpatient clinic services also commenced at a popular mission-owned secondary health care facility in Abeokuta called Sacred Heart Hospital, Lantoro, Abeokuta.

The establishment of the 'Hope Villa', an 11-room purpose built warden-supervised transitional rehabilitation hostel and group home for patients discharged from the hospital, in preparation for independent community life was another opening up strategy. The hostel is located in the vicinity of the Lantoro annexe of the hospital and a segment of the structure serves as the day-centre.

Sheltered vocational training (apprenticeship) arrangements have been made with artisans in various vocations such barbing, shoe making, vulcanizing, information and communication technologies (ICT) in the community for the training placements of long-stay patients in the rehabilitation ward, as well as discharged patients. Community assessment treatment services (CATS) were also established for domiciliary care in the community. Services rendered include assessment, treatment and transfer to the hospital when necessary, and these can be accessed through personal or telephone requests to the overall nursing supervisor on duty.

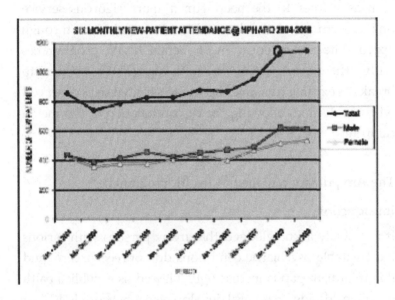

Figure 1. Patient attendance at Neuropsychiatric Hospital, Aro, 2004-2008.

Impact of the programmes

Increased service utilisation was observed in the hospital since the commencement of the community programmes and especially during the period of the television mental health education phone-in programme between July - December 2007 and January - June 2008. The increase in service use peaked and started to decline six months following the discontinuation of television programme. The service catchment area of the hospital also became more defined with the community enlightenment as the percentage of clients from Ogun State steadily increased in comparison with residents of other states .

The observed changes in service utilisation pattern was seen as pointer to the need for a more rigorous service delivery to a defined catchment population through appropriate implementation of mental health programmes within the existing primary health care (PHC) services, to break the existing dynamic barriers to service use as observed with the decline following the discontinuation of the media campaign.

The Aro primary care mental health programme

Introduction

It is globally acknowledged that many persons with serious but treatable psychiatric conditions do not receive care, and this treatment gap is increasingly viewed as a public health issue worldwide. In several developing countries only 10% or less of patients with psychiatric disorders access treatment. Service provision at PHC level has been recommended by WHO to close this gap[1,2] and the rationale includes, improved access, stigma reduction, better treatment outcome, community integration, and reduction in rights abuse associated with institutional care, as well as capacity building for mental health.

Programme Objectives

    i.   To collaborate with relevant stakeholders for effective integration of mental health service into PHC in all 20 LGAs of Ogun state Nigeria.

ii.   To train PHC workers to deliver priority mental health service.

iii. To provide essential materials, and continuing specialist support and supervision for trained PHC workers.

iv.   To establish a backup community mental health service for referrals and follow-ups.

v.   To establish a framework for continuing programme evaluation, improvement and sustainability.

Integration process and procedures

1. Pilot phase launched on 16th February 2010, at two health centres in Abeokuta North Local Government Area.

2. Planning of the state-wide extension mid-2010, with a

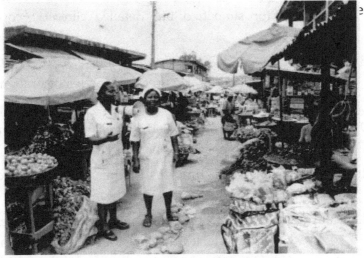

Figure 2. Primary health care workers in the community.

3. Partnerships with the University of Manchester and Lancashire Care National Health Service (NHS) Foundation Trust, United Kingdom under a British Council's Health-Links scheme.

4. Collaboration with the State Ministry of Health, Local Government Service Commission; Primary Care Development Board; PHC heads of 20 LGAs in the state.

5. Each local government area (LGA) nominated 4 PHC workers and selected 2 PHC centres (urban & rural) for the programme.

6. Local contextualisation of the WHO mhGAP intervention guide was carried out, consisting of assessment flow charts and treatment/referral guidelines for 5 priority conditions: (psychosis, depression, epilepsy, other significant emotional complaints (OSEC), mental neurological substance use disorder).

7. Design of case record sheets for each of the five priority conditions for simplified but detailed clinical record keeping.

8. Development of a 3-day training course for the PHC workers, consisting of lectures, video demonstrations clips, discussions and role-plays.

9. Training sessions were carried out in locations within each of the 4 socio-political zones of Ogun State.

10. The effectiveness and impact of training was evaluated through pre and post assessment of trainees.[3]

11. State launching of programme on 10th October 2011—World Mental Health Day. With distribution of programme materials: drugs, community mental health

mobilisation posters and handbills, and 3-month state-wide radio broadcast of programme jingle for public awareness.

12. Service delivery by the 80 trained PHC workers supported and supervised by 8 zonal field supervisors (trained experienced psychiatric nurses) by telephone and fortnightly visit. The supervisors also carry out community outreach activities.

13. Referral consultations carried out by 4 field consultants at designated PHC centres in each of the 4 zones of the state.

14. Monthly review of programme by implementation committee for programme monitoring, evaluation and improvements. We are currently adopting the QI model of the Institute for Healthcare Improvement (IHI) US, for service improvement.

Results

12 month service output and outcome

There were 473 patients who assessed the service and who were managed at 40 PHC centres in the state over a 12-month period. Almost two-thirds (60%) experienced greater than 30% symptom reduction since the first presentation and 42% had at least 2-point increase in their global rating of subjective well-being since first presentation.

12 Months Service Output Measures (Nov. 2011- Oct 2012

Zones	Trained Health Workers	Total Cases	Diagnostic Breakdown of Cases				
			Psychosis	Depression	Epilepsy	OSEC	SUD
Egba	16	120	52	12	51	3	2
Remo	17	104	54	7	38	4	1
Yewa	13	117	53	9	48	5	2
Ijebu	15	132	58	20	44	3	7
Total	61	473	217 (45.9%)	48 (10.1%)	181 (38.3%)	15 (3.2%)	12 (2.5%)

Figure 3.

47 Months Service Output Measures (Nov. 2011- Sept. 2015)

ZONES	TOTAL CASES No.	Diagnostic Breakdown of Cases					New/F.Up cases in Sept.2015
		Psychosis	Depression	Epilepsy	OSEC	Sub. Use Disorder	
EGBA	410	179	23	201	5	2	8/84
REMO	301	133	28	132	6	2	7/63
YEWA	404	207	25	161	9	2	7/86
IJEBU	457	185	67	180	10	15	5/115
ALL	1572	704 (44.8)	143 (9.1)	674 (42.9)	30 (1.9)	21 (1.3)	27/348

Figure 4.

Discussion, lessons and challenges

There was evidence of improved access to MHS in the state and service utilisation mainly for obvious conditions. Depression and substance use disorders appear to be hidden morbidities at the primary care level. However the programme's ability to provide effective intervention with minimum referral for these conspicuous 'level 3' mental health morbidities at the PHC[4] is a major feat.

There has been a remarkable impact of service as revealed by the proportion of clients with significant symptom reduction and improved subjective well-being rating. The latter addressing current emphasis on reported outcome by the service users at consultations. A good proportion of the patients also remained in treatment. Intensive supervision was needed to drive and sustain service and this may have contributed to the high rate of attrition of trained PHC workers.

The success of the programme and its sustainability are attributed to the following factors: strong professional and institutional commitment; successful partnerships; inter-agency collaborations and boundary negotiations; a solid framework for continuing support and supervision; and the supply of affordable medication and materials; solution to problems of regular transfer of LG health workers; top up training for PHC workers to sustain knowledge and skills; and supplementary training of additional staff to correct attrition.

The hospital community mental health programme would have required the mobilisation of the insufficient hospital-based professionals into the community. The solution to which was the adoption of the task shifting approach of training non-mental health professionals to provide the service under on-going supervision and support. Of the five priority conditions addressed, psychosis, depression and epilepsy constituted 96% of cases seen and successfully treated at the health centres. Cases of depression seen and treated had consistently remained at about 10% less than psychosis (44%) and epilepsy (42%). This finding suggests the hidden and possibly camouflaged nature of depression at the community and Primary Health Care (CPH) level.

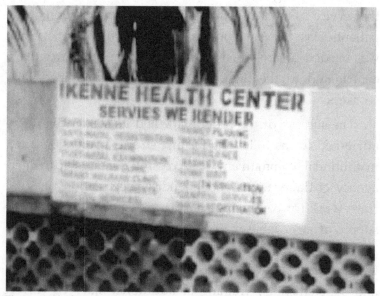

Figure 4. Signboards advertising the services offered are useful for prospective clients.

One of the most exciting aspects of the innovation is successful negotiation of the barriers between tertiary health care and the primary health care management structures for a mutually beneficial collaborative work at the PHC level. The programme supervisors, have over time, acquired the skill of supervising health workers over which they do not have formal control. This is a scenario of leading across boundaries. The programme has also opened opportunities for community mobilisation and engagement for mental health service delivery in very remote rural communities of the state. Special enlightenment programmes have been mounted for depression awareness and recognition at community level, as well as the retraining of the programme PHC workers to address the low presentation and recognition of depression at PHC.

Impact

Since programme inception five years back, the rate of service use has not declined despite challenges of human recourse attrition necessitating additional task for the programme supervisors who had to assume care-provider roles in certain centres until replacement of trained PHC workers lost to either retirement, resignations, transfers, promotion to other schedules. Participants in the programme remained proud and passionate about the service been rendered. The programme is gaining more state, national and international recognition as an efficient model for appropriate mental health service delivery at grassroots level. It is very encouraging and exciting to find rural health centres proudly including mental health service among services they provide on their signages. This shows we are winning the war against stigma.

What's next?

Service expansion is required in the area of increasing the number of trained health workers and number of participating treatment centres for mental health services delivery. Top-up training is also needed for the trained health workers especially for depression assessment and recognition. The barriers to these had been human resource shortage at the PHC, and funding limitations for additional training. We are encouraging the local government service commission to recruit additional health personnel to boost primary health care service in the state.

People with depression are not readily recognised by family and community members, compared with individuals with psychosis or epilepsy, and hence do not often readily present for orthodox care. When they do, they are likely to present with other bodily complaints which makes their recognition rather difficult for the trained primary care health workers. The proof of this is that when we applied quality improvement methodology to enhance recognition of depression among all patients presenting at PHC, through testing the idea of routine screening for depression by all PHC workers, apart from those trained to carry out mental health care. The 2-week test yielded significant improvement in the recognition and management of depression, but the routine screening for all patients by all PHC workers was unsustainable because of workload complaints resulting from human resource shortages.

References

1. World Health Organization (1978). *Mental disorders: glossary and guide to their classification in accordance with the 9th revision of the International Classification of Diseases.* Geneva: WHO

2. World Health Organization (2008). *Mental Health Gap Action Programme (mhGAP): scaling up care for mental, neurological and substance abuse disorders.* Geneva: WHO

3. Adebowale T, Onofa LU, Gater R, Akinhanmi A, Ogunlesi A, Helme C, Wood G, Ibikunle I. (2014). Evaluation of a Mental Health Training Course for Primary Health Care Workers in Ogun State, South West, Nigeria. *J Psychiatry* 17: 5.

4. Goldberg D, Huxley P. (1980). *Mental Illness in the Community: the pathway to psychiatric care.* London: Tavistock Publications

Other selected readings

Adebowale T, Onofa LU, Ighoroje M, Richard G, Ogunwale A, Okewole N, Ogundele A, Olarinde S, Olaitan F, Ogunyomi K. (2017). Experience of Trained Primary Health Care Workers in Mental Health Service Delievery Across Ogun State Nigeria. *Clin Psychiatry,* 3:1.

Aro Primary Care Mental Health programme on Mental Health Innovation Network–http://mhinnovation.net/innovations/aro-primary-care-mental-health-programme#

Cheryl A. (2017). A Nigerian hospital tackles mental illness. *Global Healthcare Insights Magazine* - International coverage of hospitals and health systems. https://globalhealthi.com

page 74 is blank

5

Psychiatric Disorders in Pregnant and Postpartum Women

Abiodun Abioye and Bode Williams

Abstract

Psychiatric disorders are a leading cause of death and complications in women during pregnancy and after childbirth. Currently, there is an increasing global awareness of the adverse impact of perinatal mental health disorders (PNMHD) on women's physical health, reproductive health, family, social and work life. Additionally, the children of women with mental health issues are more likely to suffer physical abuse, violence, death; develop abnormal cognitive and behavioural developmental problems.

The exact prevalence of PNMHD in sub-Saharan African (SSA) women is not known. There are currently no ideal screening tools. Additionally, discriminatory cut-off points for diagnosing PNMHD in affected and non-affected women are yet to be established in local studies. It has been estimated that approximately 15-40% of SSA women experience psychiatric disorders during pregnancy and after childbirth compared with 10-15% of women in high-income countries. Also, the impact and burden of mental health illness is greater in women in low income countries. This is confounded by poverty, poor social and nutritional status, reduced availability of trained healthcare professionals and inadequately resourced health care facilities.

Keywords: Post-partum; psychosis; multidisciplinary team; education; family

Introduction

Postpartum psychosis is a heterogenous condition. Women are at an increased risk of developing psychosis immediately after childbirth. The symptoms occur rapidly and include bizarre behaviour, confusion, hallucinations and delusions. These women require immediate hospitalization and urgent treatment because of the increased risk of suicides and infanticides.

In this chapter, there is a brief overview of the epidemiology in Nigerian literature. The pathogenesis, clinical features, risk assessment and management of postpartum psychosis are also discussed.

Epidemiology: overview of Nigerian literature

Pregnancy-related psychiatric disorder has been an important field of study for decades due to the range, specific risk issues, and impact on maternal welfare and child safety and development. Mental disorders linked to pregnancy cannot be comprehensively looked at without reviewing the psychiatric illnesses in young females, the psychological, psychiatric and pharmacological issues in pregnancy, and postpartum psychiatric disorders.

In Nigeria and other African states, several studies have looked at epidemiological factors and possible aetiological factors, with clinical management being essentially similar in all settings. Clinical features are similar, but most diagnostic tools used in African settings have been adapted locally. The International Classification of Diseases and Related Health Problems (ICD 10)[1] and the Diagnostic and Statistical Manual of Mental Disorders (DSM 5)[2] take account of variable presentations in various populations when defining diagnostic criteria.

Sulyman used the Edinburgh postnatal depression scale on 483 women in a maternity unit in northeastern Nigeria.[3] They noted a postnatal depression rate of 22.4%. Possible risk factors included unemployment, lack of support from partners, primiparity, unplanned pregnancy and maternal physical illness. Sawyer et al. identified in a systematic review of the literature that depression was the most commonly identified perinatal psychiatric disorder, with a prevalence of 11.3% during pregnancy and 18.3% after birth.[4] Anxiety disorders were next with 14.8% in pregnancy and 14.0% after birth. Post-traumatic stress disorder (PTSD) had a prevalence of 5.9% after birth.

Uwakwe et al. used the postnatal depression scale and the Zung self-rating depression scale to screen all postpartum women at the Nnamdi Azikiwe University Teaching Hospital, Nigeria.[5] They also conducted the structured interview schedule of the CIDI and the affective module of the ICD10 symptom checklist. From a total of 225 women, 24 (10.7%) subjects met the strict diagnostic criteria for depressive disorders.

Other studies that looked at epidemiology include the one by Danasabe and Elias.[6] They used the Edinburgh postnatal depression scale to screen 175 Hausa mothers for depression. The Edinburgh postnatal depression scale is a well-validated 10-item questionnaire commonly used to screen for clinical depression. The total score is determined by summing up together the scores of each of the items.

Scores of 10 and above indicate the presence of clinical depression, with higher scores indicating more severe depressive symptoms. They reported a prevalence of 36% using a strict cut-off score of 12, but higher rates with a less stringent score. Cut off scores that were considered ranged from 10 (which had a prevalence of 45.7%) to 13 (which had a prevalence of 28.0%).

Associated factors in their study included marital status (single, divorced or married status), unemployment and mode of delivery (unassisted vaginal deliveries or operative deliveries). The rates of depression were found to be higher in divorced women (57.6%) compared to married women (39.8%). Likewise, 26.3% of the unemployed respondents had depression compared to 6.9% of unemployed respondents. The mode of delivery was documented to have a statistically significant association, with 14 out of 24 rated as depressed, but comparative rates for women with normal deliveries was not given.

Ndukuba et al also confirmed the high psychiatric morbidity in Nigerian mothers.[7] In their retrospective case note study of women diagnosed with postpartum psychiatric conditions in a federal neuropsychiatric hospital in Enugu between 2009 and 2011, they found high rates of schizophrenic disorders (48.7%) and depression (22%) based on the ICD10 diagnostic criteria. Furthermore, most patients in this cohort were between 20 and 30 years old. Additionally, there was a higher rate of psychiatric disorders in women from the rural areas. A difference in rate of peripartum pyschiatric disorders between rural and urban dwellers has not been previously reported in other studies.

Overall, schizophrenia (48.7%) appeared to be the most common severe psychiatric condition that required care within tertiary facilities in this population.

Postpartum psychosis

In his article titled: "Perinatal Psychiatric Disorders," in the Royal College of Psychiatrist's textbook, *Seminars in Adult Psychiatry*, George Stein classified perinatal psychiatric disorders into three groups:[8]

i.   **Postpartum psychosis**: This is a rare, severe and life threatening illness which complicates 2 per 2000 deliveries.

ii. **Postnatal anxiety-depressive related disorders**: This category includes conditions such as panic disorders, anxiety and obsessional disorders, and affects 10% of women. The symptoms usually manifest immediately after childbirth.

iii. **Maternity (postpartum) blues**: This condition is considered to be a normal reaction to childbirth and affects 50% of women. It is not a clinical disorder.

A fourth group of disorders is bonding difficulties, which can result in child abuse. This tends to have a multi-factorial aetiology that requires assessment and input by perinatal psychiatrists. The rest of this article will focus on the pathogenesis, clinical features, risk assessment and management of postpartum psychosis.

Puerperal psychosis, otherwise known as postpartum psychosis, has its clinical and diagnostic features defined in standard psychiatric textbooks. It is actually a range of psychiatric disorders as defined in the International Classification of Diseases (ICD 10),[1] but it does have certain peculiar features that make it quite distinct. The ICD 10 assumes that puerperal mental illnesses are not distinguishable from mood disorders and psychotic (mainly schizophrenic) disorders, but in situations where they cannot be properly classified, the diagnosis of 'mental and behavioural disorder associated with the puerperium, not otherwise classified' is given.

Clinical features

In the DSM 5[2], there are specifiers for peripartum onset mood disorders and peripartum onset depressive disorders within the affective disorders and depressive disorders section of that widely-used *American Psychiatric Association Manual.* Classically, it is said to have an abrupt onset usually emerging from day three after childbirth, but can occur at anytime up to six months. Notable early signs include restless activity, disinhibition, fleeting anger and negativistic behaviour, profound insomnia, anxiety and a state of fear. A state of delirium tends to help differentiate it from maternity blues.

Karnosh and Hope gave a classic description that remains relevant.[9] It was described as "panic, sudden aversion and distrust of relatives, misidentification, hallucinosis, sing-song chat, poor affect and elevated temperature." Women with postpartum psychosis frequently experience psychotic symptoms, including delusions that the infant is possessed, as well as 'command hallucinations' to kill the infant. However, these psychotic symptoms are not universal.

Two French physicians, Jean Esquirol and Louis Victor Marce, carefully described the clinical features of 100 women with postpartum psychosis in the 19th century. They outlined the basic clinical features of the disorder(s) that were used as a reference in the various diagnostic instruments that were designed later.

The DSM 5 states that the peripartum onset specifier for both bipolar and depressive episodes can be used if the onset of mood symptoms occur during pregnancy or within 4 weeks after delivery. In women presenting with postpartum mental health disorders, it is paramount to differentiate between pyschotic symptoms and delirium during clinical evaluation. In general, postpartum mood episodes with psychotic features complicate between 1 in 500 deliveries and 1 in 1000 deliveries, and there is a higher prevalence among primiparous women. Women with personal and/or family history of mood disorders are at increased risk. The risk of recurrence in subsequent pregnancies is between 30% to 50%. Frank schizophrenic and schizo-affective disorders have also been described in the postpartum period.

Pathogenesis

Neuroendocrine dysfunction and psycho-social factors have been implicated as potential causative factors in postpartum psychosis. It has been hypothesised that the sharp decline in oestrogen after delivery may be contributory to postpartum psychosis. Some authors have postulated that the sharp drop in progesterone (30- fold drop), increased cortisol levels (one study reported significantly elevated post-dexamethasone cortisol levels in women with postpartum psychosis) and disturbances in thyroid hormone concentrations are contributory factors. All these hormonal changes are known to have an impact on the mood by affecting a number of neurotransmitters in the brain that control mood changes.[10] Oestrogen drop after childbirth may expose dopamine receptors which have been rendered supersensitive by high levels of oestrogen during pregnancy. High cortisol levels are frequently associated with depressive disorders and dysphoria, which are well recognized clinical features of Cushing's syndrome.

During the postpartum period, 10% of women develop hypothyroidism due to a sharp decline in thyroid hormone concentrations after delivery. It is well-recognized that women with postpartum hypothyroidism can exhibit psychiatric symptoms. There is a well-known overlap between the manifestations of thyroid disorders and psychiatric illnesses. They can trigger anxiety and mood-related symptoms. Disturbances in the hypothalamic-pituitary axis, with blunting of responses to the thyrotropin releasing hormone (TRH), have also been reported in another study as a potential factor. This is possibly by triggering transient hypothyroidism, with depression as a clinical feature.[11]

Familial factors have also been implicated in the aetiology of postpartum psychosis. In a systematic review, Thuwe analyzed pooled data from a series of ten papers published between 1911 and 1973.[12] About 614 women with postpartum pyschosis were reviewed, of these 40% had a family history of mental illness, including psychoses, affective disorders, psychopathy, alcoholism and suicide. Jones and Craddock found that a puerperal psychotic episode occurred in 74% of a cluster of 27 women with a family history of psychosis, compared to 30% without a family history.[13] In their study, childbirth was found to be a potent trigger for psychosis in women with a familial tendency to develop puerperal psychosis.

Social factors have not been found to play a major role in precipitating severe postpartum psychotic disorders. Systematic studies done in the United Kingdom did not establish any links between recent life events and postpartum depression.[14] Other studies showed that stress may increase admission rate.[15]

Management and risk issues

Psychiatric disorders are best managed with a multi-disciplinary approach. This has been adopted as standard practice in most countries. The Royal College of Psychiatrists in the United Kingdom emphasizes this approach. This basically means that the conditions are managed by clinical teams that include psychiatrists, nurses, psychologists, social workers and occupational therapists. The multi-disciplinary approach is imperative due to the need for various disciplines to have an input in the management of psychiatric disorders. The process evolved in Europe and America after the closure of the large asylums in the 1950s. This led to large reforms in the mental health services. Papers like *Modernising Mental*

Health Services and the *National Service Framework for Mental Health in the UK* are examples of recent guiding principles. The National Institute for Health and Excellence (NICE) in the UK have produced evidence-based guidelines predominantly based on systematic reviews to support the multi-disciplinary approach of the management of most psychiatric disorders.

Initial evaluation and risk assessment

Management follows a process of detailed history taking, serial mental state examinations, risk assessment, differential diagnosis and formulation. The formulation is a systematic process of having a comprehensive understanding of the patient by evaluating predisposing factors, precipitating factors and maintaining factors. The predisposing factors are usually derived from the patient's background. This will include biological/genetic factors, psychological issues from childhood and social factors. Similarly, precipitating (usually stressful events) and maintaining factors (ongoing issues like relationship/family problems, drug use and social issues like finances and housing) should be identified during initial assessment using systematic multi-modal approach.

A thorough general and systemic physical examination should be performed. Routine blood screening studies, including full blood count, ESR/ CRP, random blood sugar levels, renal function tests, liver function tests and thyroid function test should be requested. In some cases, specialized neuroendocrine studies may be required. These tests are important for diagnosis and will exclude secondary causes of delirium.

Risk assessment and the use of diagnostic tools like the PANSS (for psychosis), Beck's depression scale and the structured clinical interview schedule for DSM 5 disorders are all potentially useful tools for documenting accurate diagnosis. Suicide risk assessments and violence risk assessments can be done with tools such as the Short Term Assessment of Risk and Treatability (START). The HCR20 is useful in patients with a past history of violent conduct. Singh et al identified about 10 useful violent risk assessment tools for schizophrenia and other psychiatric disorders.[16]

Treatment options

An individualized treatment and care plan is usually recommended. The type of treatment required should be tailored to individual needs. The level of care offered is dependent on the score on risk assessment and the availability of resources at the local units. Inpatient care, home treatment, outpatient care and day hospital facilities are all possible options in different settings. There are mother and baby inpatient facilities in the UK, but they are not commonly used elsewhere. Pharmacological treatment targets specific diagnostic categories, antipsychotics and mood stabilizing agents. Antidepressants and electro-convulsive therapy are indicated in moderate to severe depressive disorders. Electroconvulsive therapy (ECT) is known to be highly effective in psychotic depression, severe suicidal states and intractable mania.

Psychotropic medications during pregnancy and lactation

Antipsychotic medications are usually considered as first-line treatment for postpartum psychosis. The effect of many antipsychotic medications on newborn and infant development is not known as there are no randomized controlled trials on pregnant women. All psychotropic medications are excreted into the breast milk and transferred to the infant. The benefit of medication should be weighed against the risks for each individual prior to treatment. On balance, women with postpartum psychosis should be encouraged to continue breastfeeding if they wish, as this might improve compliance during treatment.

The choice of antipsychotics should be restricted to medications with a good safety profile during pregnancy and lactation. Hence, quetiapine, olanzapine and risperidone are considered as first-line treatment, as they have a better safety data. The decision to introduce conventional antipsychotropic medications such as haloperidol, trifluoperazine and thiothixene should be made on a case-by-case basis, as there is limited information about the safety of these medications during pregnancy and breastfeeding.

Benzodiazipines such as lorazepam and clonazepam can be used in conjunction with antipsychotropics to control agitation and promote sleeping during the initial stages of treatment. There is, however, very limited safety information and there are no controlled trials on the use of benzo-diazipine during pregnancy and lactation (table 1). It is recommended that treatment should continue for at least 12 months after clinical remission to reduce the risk of a relapse.

Table 1. Summary of the teratogenic effects and adverse neonatal effects of psychotropic medications

Medication	Potential fetal and newborn effects
Tricyclic antidepressants	• No reports of congenital malformation • Possible transient withdrawal symptoms in neonates • Respiratory depression has been reported with doxepin, but others are deemed safe
SSRIs	• Very commonly used in pregnancy • No evidence of congenital malformations • Transient apnoea has been reported with citalopram during lactation
Antipsychotics	• Floppy infant syndrome and other minor anomalies have been reported with clozapine but with limited information on significant harm with other atypical antipsychotics • Typical antipsychotics have been used for over 40 years. Sparse data linking them to teratogenic or toxic effects, but doses should be minimized
Mood stabilizers	• Valproate should be avoided in pregnancy as there are associations with neural tube defects, craniofacial anomalies and cardiac defects. It may be better tolerated durng breast feeding • Carbamazepine and Lithium are also teratogenic. There is limited data on teratogenic effects for other mood stabilizers. High strength preconceptual folate supplements (5mg, once daily) are recommended with lamotrigine.
Benzodiazepines	• Neonatal sedation, withdrawal symptoms, neurocognitive effects and toxicity may occur during breastfeeding.

Electroconvulsive therapy

Electroconvulsive therapy should be considered in patients who are unreponsive to, or who cannot tolerate psychotropic medications. It has the strongest evidence for bringing about rapid remission in severe affective illnesses (mania and depression), but the effect tends to be short-lived and the treatment has a poor reputation with the public. Most of its action is not totally clear, but it is linked to altering the expressions and functions of neurotransmitters linked to psychiatric disorders. This includes dopamine, serotonin, and others like gamma-amino butyric acid (GABA) and glutamate. They also have effects on the hypothalamic-pituitary-adrenal axis (HPA axis). The ECT is still in use, but strictly regulated in most Western settings. In the UK, guidelines for its use have been issued by various bodies including the Royal College of Psychiatrists (College Report CR176).

Psychosocial interventions

Psychological treatment includes cognitive behavioural therapy (CBT) and supportive therapies. Dialectical behavioural therapy (DBT) can also be used as an adjunctive therapy once acute depressive and psychotic symptoms have been controlled. These treatment modalities have been shown to be effective in patients with comorbid borderline personality disorders and postnatal depressive illnesses. Psychologists play an important role. They should be involved during initial risk assessment and during the follow-up assessment of mother-child interaction. Psychologists also have a central role in the management of comorbid issues like insomnia, anxiety disorders and interpersonal and social difficulties. Social care, occupational therapy and intensive nursing input in all settings are essential parts of the multi-disciplinary approach. Other aspects of management include liaison with obstetricians and childcare services, and ensuring smooth communication.

Education of patient and family members

Education is a key aspect of prevention. The patient, their partners and close relatives should be educated on how to recognize the early symptoms and signs of psychosis, and seek prompt medical intervention.

Consequences and relapses

Women with psychosis are more likely to commit infanticide, suicide, child abuse and neglect compared with the background population. As an example, Jennings et al, found that up to 41% of depressed mothers with children under age 3 had thoughts of harming a child compared to 7% of a control group.[17] These women are also more likely to develop chronic psychiatric disorders, relapses in subsequent pregnancies, substance abuse and have impaired functional deficits.

Summary and conclusion

- Postpartum psychosis is a medical emergency.
- Early recognition of symptoms and signs of psychosis and prompt treatment are key to management.
- Cases should be managed by experienced multidisciplinary teams skilled in the management of postpartum psychosis.

- Treatment should be individualized and tailored according to the needs and availability of resources at local treatment centres.

- Education of the patient and family members is important in preventing relapse.

Learning points and objectives

- Medical emergency
- Early recognition of symptoms and prompt treatment
- Multidisciplinary management
- Education of the family members is important in prevention

References

1. WHO. *The ICD-10 Classification of Mental and Behavioural Disorders: Clinical Descriptions and Diagnostic Guidelines.* World Health Organization, Geneva. 1992

2. American Psychiatric Association. *Diagnostic and Statistical Manual of Mental Disorders.* 5th edition American Psychiatric Association, Washington, 2013.

3. Sulyman D, Ayanda KA, Dattijo LM, Aminu BM. Postnatal depression and its associated factors among northeastern Nigerian women. *Annals of Tropical Medicine and Public Health* 2016; 9(3): 184-190.

4. Sawyer A, Ayers S, Smith H. Pre-and postnatal psychological well-being in Africa: A systematic review. *Journal of Affective Disorders* 2010; 123(1): 17-29.

5. Uwakwe R. Affective (depressive) morbidity in puerperal Nigerian women: Validation of the Edinburgh Postnatal Depression Scale. *Acta Psychiatrica Scandinavica* 2003; 107(4): 251-9.

6. Danasabe M, Elias NB. Postpartum depression among Hausa ethnic women in Abubakar Tafawa Balewa University Teaching Hospital, northeast Nigeria. *International Journal of Research in Humanities, Arts and Literature* 2016; 14(3): 55-64.

7. Ndukuba AC, Odinka PC, Muomah RC, Nwoha SO. Clinical and socio-demographic profile of women with post-partum psychiatric conditions at a federal neuropsychiatric hospital in southeast Nigeria between 2009 and 2011. *Annals of Medical and Health Sciences Research* 2015; 5(3): 168-72.

8. Stein G. Perinatal psychiatric disorders, p. 635-664. In Stein G, Wilkinson G, editors, *Seminars in General Adult Psychiatry*. Second Edition. Royal College of Psychiatrists, UK,, 2007.

9. Karnosh LJ, Hope JM. Puerperal psychoses and their sequelae. *American Journal of Psychiatry* 1937; 94, 537-550.

10. Wieck A. Ovarian hormones, mood and neurotransmitters. *International Review of Psychiatry* 1996; 8(1): 17-25.

11. Ijuin T, Douchi T, Yamamoto S, Ijuin Y, Nagata Y. The relationship between maternity blues and thyroid dysfunction. *Journal of Obstetrics and Gynaecology Research* 1998; 24(1): 49-55.

12. Thuwe I. Genetic factors in puerperal psychosis. *British Journal of Psychiatry* 1974; 125: 378-385.

13. Jones I, Craddock N. Familiality of the puerperal trigger in bipolar disorder: Results of a family study. *American Journal of Psychiatry* 2001; 158, 913- 917.

14. Dowlatshahi D, Paykel ES. Life events and social stress in puerperal psychoses: Absence of effect. *Psychological Medicine* 1990; 20(3): 655-62.

15. Allwood CW, Berk M, Bodemer W. An investigation into puerperal psychoses in black women admitted to Baragwanath Hospital. *South African Medical Journal* 2000; 90(5), 518-520

16. Singh JP, Serper M, Reinharth J, Fazel S. Structured assessment of violence risk in schizophrenia and other psychiatric disorders: A systematic review of the validity, reliability, and item content of 10 available instruments. *Schizophrenia Bulletin* 2011; 37(5): 899-912.

17. Jennings KD, Ross S, et al. Thoughts of harming infants in depressed and non-depressed mothers. *J Affective Disorders* 1999; 54:21-28.

6
Changing Landscape of Child and Adolescent Mental Health in sub-Saharan Africa

Olayinka Omigbodun, Kwabena Kusi-Mensah
Tolulope Bella-Awusah, Cornelius Ani

Abstract

This chapter discusses child and adolescent mental health (CAMH), emphasising the developmental approach appropriate for this period. Narratives are also given of family, school and community factors that act as risk and protective factors for CAMH. Risk factors for CAMH problems, such as poverty, low school enrolment rates, poor educational quality and obstetric care are prevalent in sub-Saharan Africa (SSA). Gains were made with addressing these problems in SSA towards the end of the MDG era in 2015, but SSA still fell short of meeting the targets. The history of CAMH in SSA highlights a lack of focused CAMH programmes until a decade ago and the role of the International Association for Child and Adolescent Psychiatry and Allied Professions (IACAPAP) as a catalyst for CAMH in SSA, leading to the establishment of the African Association for CAMH. The few epidemiological studies on CAMH in SSA reveal similar rates as found in Western studies with 1 in every 5 children or adolescents having a CAMH problem. Studies also reveal strong negative attitudes towards CAMH problems as well as misunderstandings. Numerous social and cultural problems impacting CAMH are brought to the fore. Policies that will encourage CAMH promotion such as opportunities for positive involvement in family and school life and environments that encourage the constructive use of leisure in SSA are urgently required. The WHO Mental Health Action

Plan, SDGs, Rights of the Child and University of Ibadan Centre for CAMH all have a role to play in the transformation of CAMH in SSA.

Keywords: Child and adolescent mental health; sub-Saharan Africa; Risk and protective factors; SDGs; CRC, CCAMH, research agenda

Definitions and descriptions of child and adolescent mental health

In the World Health Organization's (WHO) Comprehensive Mental Health Action Plan — 2013 to 2020, mental health is defined as a

> . . . *state of well-being in which the individual realizes his or her own abilities, can cope with the normal stresses of life, can work productively and fruitfully, and is able to make a contribution to his or her community* (WHO, 2013).[1]

Emphasizing a developmental approach, child and adolescent mental health (CAMH) is described as an

> . . . optimal psychological development and functioning, a positive sense of self, the ability of the child or adolescent to manage his/her thoughts, emotions and build social relationships, the aptitude to learn and acquire an education and the opportunity to ultimately be able to have full participation in the society (WHO et al., 2005, WHO, 2013).[2,1]

This description reflects the growth and development that occur during this critical period of life. Other descriptions of CAMH by WHO further highlight family, school and community as key areas that impact the mental health of children and adolescents (WHO, 2005).[3] The risk and protective factors for the mental health of children and adolescents are summarized in table 1 below.

Table 1. Selected mental health risk and protective factors in the family, school and community

Domain	Risk Factors	Protective Factors
Family	• Inconsistent care-giving • Family conflict • Poor family discipline ▪ Poor family management ▪ Death of a family member	▪ Family attachment ▪ Opportunities for positive involvement in the family ▪ Authoritative parenting with good boundary setting and nurturing
School	▪ Academic failure ▪ Failure of schools to provide an appropriate environment to support attendance and learning ▪ Bullying and victimisation ▪ Inadequate or inappropriate educational provision	▪ Opportunities for involvement in school life ▪ Positive reinforcement for academic achievement ▪ Positive identity with school and need for educational attainment ▪ Supportive and nurturing educational strategies
Community	▪ Community disorganization	▪ Connectedness to community ▪ Opportunities for

Domain	Risk Factors	Protective Factors
	■ Discriminati on and marginalizati on ■ Exposure to violence ■ Lack of sense of place in the society ■ Transitions such as urbanisation	constructive use of leisure ■ Positive cultural experiences ■ Positive role models ■ Rewards for community involvement ■ Connection with positive c o m m u n i t y organizations including religious organizations ■ Social, cultural, and economic policies that promote fairness and equity

Adapted from the World Health Organisation (WHO, 2005)[3]

The importance of home, school and community impacts on the mental health of children and adolescents described arlier in the seminal work of Sameroff and colleagues[4] cannot be overstated. Risk factors such as poverty, parental drug abuse and mental illness, parental low educational attainment or its absence, child abuse in the family, exposure to racism and large family size were examined in relation to cognitive functioning. When none of these factors was present in a child, the average Intelligence Quotient (IQ) of a child was 119. With one risk factor, the average IQ dropped to 116; with two risk factors, it dropped to 113 and with four and eight risk factors, it dropped to 93 and 85 respectively as seen in figure 1 below.

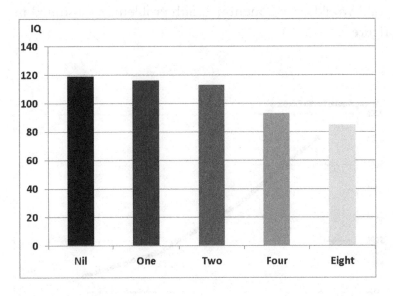

Figure 1. Impact of mental health risk factors on intelligence quotient of children and adolescents (Sameroff et al)[4]

Sameroff and colleagues[4] also looked at the opportunities to improve the mental health of children and the effect of an accumulation of opportunities. These opportunities were referred to as assets. Assets were drawn from the child, family, school and community. Child assets included temperament such as "child is optimistic about the future", while family assets included positive family life such as "family life provides high level of support". School assets included a "supportive and caring school environment", while community assets were "peaceful and clean neighbourhoods", or "positive role models for children in the community". The more assets a child had, the less likely the child would have a mental health problem as illustrated in figure 2.

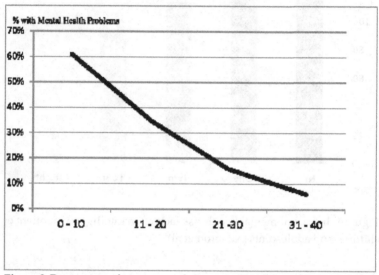

Figure 2. Percentage of young people in mental health problem category versus assets possessed.[4]

Of the children with 31- 40 assets, 6% were in the mental health problem category, for children with 21-30 assets, 16% were in the mental health problem category, of the children with 11-20 assets, 35% were in the mental health problem category, and for those with 0-10 assets, almost two-thirds (61%) were in the mental health problem category.

Of the factors identified in Sameroff's paper, poverty remains a major problem in sub-Saharan Africa as indicated by the failure to meet the recently ended Millennium Development Goals, specifically goal 1: *the halving of poverty by 2015* (UN, 2015).[5] Education and school environment or enrolment issues are still major problems with sub-Saharan Africa (SSA), again failing to meet the MDG 2 targets (UN, 2015).[5] Despite improvements in CAMH in most countries in SSA as a result of working towards the Millennium Development Goals (MDGs) (UN, 2015)[5], there are still problems of poor obstetric care with perinatal injuries, problems with childhood nutrition and other aetiological factors for mental health problems. At the close of the era of MDGs, SSA still had the highest child mortality rates, but also the highest absolute decline in child mortality rates (UN, 2015).[5]

More and more children in SSA are surviving beyond infancy after traumatic obstetric processes which lead to mental health problems that manifest later in life.[6] There is therefore a need for an urgent review of CAMH in SSA and urgent steps to be put in place to address the evident gaps. The World Health Organisation (WHO) admitted that due to a focus on childhood mortality, planning for CAMH suffered neglect worldwide.[7] In reality, CAMH has only begun to receive concerted attention in the last decade.

A brief history of child and adolescent mental health in sub-Saharan Africa (SSA)

The absence of any explicit mental health-related goals in the MDGs is a reflection of the lack of prioritization of mental health. The earliest documentation of CAMH professionals coming together in sub-Saharan Africa was in Khartoum, Sudan in 1972 during the 3rd Pan-African Psychiatric Congress. In a write up on the development of mental health services for children in the African region, Olatawura[8] mentioned that the Khartoum meeting gave professionals from different parts of Africa an opportunity to share their experiences with children with various neuropsychiatric conditions, but no mention was made of planning to meet again or to form a body. Until a little over a decade ago, there was virtually no focus on CAMH in sub-Saharan Africa. Only South Africa and Tunisia had planned and established services for child psychiatry, and South Africa was the only country on the continent with formal training facilities for child and adolescent mental health specialists.[9]

In the last decade, the International Association for Child and Adolescent Psychiatry and Allied Professions (IACAPAP) concentrated its efforts in sub-Saharan Africa by supporting two study groups with the aim of promoting the development of effective and sustainable CAMH care.[10] Nairobi, Kenya and Abuja, Nigeria played host to the two IACAPAP supported study groups in 2007 and 2009 respectively. Facilitators and participants at these study groups have since then taken up leadership roles in CAMH in various countries in Africa, either developing services in their home regions or organising training programmes that have produced more CAMH professionals. These study groups also culminated with building up and uniting a crop of CAMH professionals, and this resulted in the establishment of the African Association for Child and Adolescent Mental Health (AACAMH) in Nairobi in 2007. This has been an important catalyst in the transformation of CAMH in Africa. Another major catalyst for change in CAMH in SSA has been the establishment of the Centre for Child and Adolescent Mental Health (CCAMH) with funding support from the John D. and Catherine T. MacArthur Foundation.[11] Before the establishment of AACAMH and CCAMH, research for CAMH in SSA was very limited.

Epidemiological studies on child and adolescent mental health in sub-Saharan Africa (SSA)

Children and adolescents constitute a third of the world's population and almost 90% live in low- and middle-income countries (LAMICs), where they form up to 50% of the population (UNICEF, 2008).[12] In spite of this, only 10% of CAMH research studies come from LAMICs[13] and an even smaller fraction from SSA. Community-based epidemiological data in most sub-Saharan countries are very few and most of the studies are either limited to hospital-based settings or have small sample sizes. However, the limited literature on community-based studies carried out in SSA does show similar rates as in Western studies with 1 in 5 children and adolescents having a mental disorder. The first epidemiological study on children's mental health in SSA was carried out among 440 Nigerians.[14] They were randomly selected from three different areas (a rural village, a low-income urban area and a more affluent area) in and around Ibadan, southwest Nigeria. The frequency of severe behavioural disorders in the whole group was 16%. The children in the low-income urban area have the highest frequency of 22%; the children in the affluent area, 14%; and the lowest rate of 11% in the rural area. Intellectual disability at 2-3% in a recent meta-analysis[15] is higher than the global average of 1%.

Attention deficit hyperactive disorder was found to have rates of 1.5% in Ethiopia and 8.7% in Nigeria,[16,17,18] Community-based studies on depression in Africa found a range of 21.2% in Nigerian adolescents[19,6,16] to as low as around 1.5% among young children with age range 6 – 15 years in Ghana[20] and Ethiopia.[18] Conduct disorder also ranged from 2% in Ghana[20] to 12.5% in Kenya.[21] Prevalence of anxiety disorders ranged from 26.6% in rural Uganda where the estimate was high presumably because of the traumatic experience of war in that area[22] to as low as 1% among primary school children in Ghana.[20] For suicidal ideation, data available from Nigeria indicates a prevalence rate of 23% of adolescents with the ideation and 12% with a previous attempt[23] with adolescents living in urban areas, coming from polygamous families, or from broken homes having higher rates.

Perceptions of and problems impacting child and adolescent mental health

Studies carried out in Nigeria reveal that there are strong negative attitudes towards people with mental disabilities.[24] Typically, the belief is that the family has either come under a curse by the gods, or is being punished for doing evil or the illness is as a result of demon-possession.[24] Another common reason is ignorance, which makes people to regard children with mental disorders as disobedient, naughty or possessed. It is within this milieu that 'spiritual healing' methods such as beatings, fasting and exorcisms appear to have flourished in Africa for mental disorders.[24] The view that spiritual forces are the cause of child and adolescent mental illness is held by many[25] and this influences help-seeking behaviour and therapy. According to Omigbodun,[25] ascribing child and adolescent mental health problems to spiritual forces could mean several things. It could mean escaping accountability—the hard work involved in changing behaviour and the responsibility for working through issues. For example, if a child having conduct problems such as stealing, lying, truancy and bullying, all probably resulting from a dysfunctional family, is labelled as being 'possessed', then the family do not give that opportunity to look inwards and see how the family life can be re-organized to provide a more stable environment for the child. The aetiology, as far as the family is concerned, remains outside of the family.

In a needs assessment for school mental health services in rural and urban southwest Nigeria, some primary school teachers expressed the view that children do not experience mental health problems, as can be seen from the quotes below.[26]—

> . . . *Emotional problems will not affect pupils because of their age. Only adults can have emotional problems. The way God created children, they don't have anything at the back of their mind that can cause much problems for them*
>
> . . . *We don't have any behavioural problems here because this place is a primary school*

Apart from negative and misguided perceptions, there are countless social problems impacting the mental health of children and adolescents living in sub-Saharan Africa, and in many instances, policy makers and country leaders show little commitment to bringing change, if any at all. Despite the fact that all countries in Africa have ratified the United Nations Convention of the Rights of the Child, there are suggestions that up to 40% of girl children in this region are married off by the age of 18.[27] Child marriages remain entrenched in African societies with the consequences of curtailed schooling and disastrous reproductive health complications which in turn lead to mental disorders for the 'child mother' and the child. With 50 million child labourers, 10 million street children, 120,000 child soldiers (a third of the world's child soldiers), over one million child sex slaves on the continent, mental health has been far from being realized for the African child.[28,3]

Studies done in Nigeria found as high as 45- 69% use of psychoactive substances[29,30] among street children in southwest Nigeria with as many as 24% working as drug couriers, almost 50% reporting to be sex-workers, and 11% admitting to being raped.[30] In northern Nigeria, the phenomenon of 'almajiri' children, a term used to describe children in northern Nigeria who are sent to live with teachers of the Qur'an by their parents to receive religious instruction is only now being explored. Due to the inability to cater for their needs, the teachers send the children to the streets to beg and carry out menial jobs.[31] A myriad of mental health challenges, including but not limited to two-thirds (66.2%) using psychoactive substance has been well documented among them.[31,32]

In addition, there are also significant psychosocial issues children and adolescents in Africa face that are inimical to their mental health. From education, poverty, physical disease to hunger and conflict, the barriers in the way of children enjoying optimum mental health are formidable. A study in southwest Nigeria revealed that problems with psychosocial stressors were present in 62.2% of children with mental health problems.[33] Psychosocial problems outlined included problems with primary support (separation from parents to live with relatives also known as extended fostering, disruption in the family, abandonment by mother, psychiatric illness in a parent) and sexual abuse, which accounted for 39.4%, as well as problems with social environment (8.7%), educational problems (30.7%) and economic problems (3.9%). Despite the myriad of identified problems, CAMH in sub-Saharan Africa is experiencing change because there are now policies and programmes driving this.

Available tools to drive the child and adolescent mental health agenda in sub-Saharan Africa

There is now available for CAMH in sub-Saharan Africa, three policy documents with a strong CAMH agenda adopted by virtually all the countries in the region. For emphasis, the documents reinforce one another with overlapping content stressing the import of CAMH. These documents might just be the way forward to move CAMH to the priority agenda in the region for peace, progress, prosperity and partnership as captured in the Sustainable Development Goals. In addition to these policy documents, working in synergy with the content of the documents is the University of Ibadan Centre for Child and Adolescent Mental

Health (CCAMH). The CAMH is experiencing rapid progress through the Mental Health Action Plan [2013 – 2020] (WHO, 2013)[1], the 2030 Agenda for Sustainable Development,[34] the United Nations Convention on the Rights of the Child[35] and the Centre for Child and Adolescent Mental Health (CCAMH).

Mental health action plan [2013 – 2020] (WHO, 2013)[1]

In May 2012, the 65th World Health Assembly (WHA) adopted resolution WHA65.4 on the global burden of mental disorders and a need for a comprehensive and coordinated response from health and social sectors at the country level. Hence in response and after consultations with member states, civil society and international partners, a mental health action plan was developed with aspects for promotion, prevention, treatment, rehabilitation and care, and recovery, with a core focus typified by the slogan: 'no health without mental health'. This has, in a very short time, contributed to the rise of CAMH globally and more specifically, in low resource regions of the world like Africa.

The mental health action plan has four main objectives as follows:

- More effective leadership and governance for mental health
- Provision of comprehensive, integrated and responsive mental health and social care services in community-based settings
- Implementation of strategies for promotion of mental health and prevention of mental disorders

- Strengthening information systems, evidence and research

For each of these objectives, there are indicators that each member state will need to monitor and give progress report on their implementation at World Health Assemblies. Likewise, each has a strong CAMH component.

Objective 1

Strengthen effective leadership and governance for mental health:

- Policies, plans and laws for mental health will comply with the United Nations Convention of the Rights of the Child (CRC)
- Inclusion and mainstreaming of mental health issues explicitly within children's health, education, disability, the judicial system, CRC, social protection, poverty reduction and development

Objective 2

Provide comprehensive, integrated and responsive mental health and social care services in community-based settings

- Health workers must be trained to attend to both the physical and mental health care needs of children and adolescents simultaneously
- Collaboration with "informal" mental health care providers, such as families and school teachers
- Provision of responsive services to women and children living with domestic violence

- Human resource development to build the knowledge and skills of general and specialized health workers to deliver evidence-based, culturally appropriate and human rights-oriented mental health and social care services for children and adolescents
- Inclusion of CAMH in undergraduate and graduate curricula

Objective 3

Implement strategies for promotion of mental health and prevention of mental health disorder

- Children and adolescents with mental disorders should be provided with early intervention through evidence-based psychosocial and other non-pharmacological interventions
- Interventions should be based in the community
- Avoid institutionalization and medicalization
- Mental health needs of children and adolescents exposed to natural disasters or civil conflict and unrest, including those who have been associated with armed forces or armed groups, are very high and require special attention

Objective 4

Strengthen information systems, evidence and research for mental health

- Data collected will be disaggregated by gender and age thereby reflecting the period of infancy, childhood and adolescence in mental health reports

Transforming our world: the 2030 agenda for sustainable development (UNDP, 2015)[34]

The Sustainable Development Agenda is a plan of action focused on 5Ps:

- Ending Poverty and Hunger for all People,
- Protecting the Planet,
- Ensuring Prosperity for all,
- Fostering Peaceful Societies, all through
- Revitalised Global Partnership for Sustainable Development.

There are 17 SDGs and over 169 targets, and unlike the MDGs, CAMH issues are rich within the agenda. Each member nation in sub-Saharan Africa needs to align with these goals and targets for rapid growth. The following SDGs can be described as CAMH SDGs because their achievement impinges directly on the focus specifically on CAMH.

Goal 1: End Poverty

It is impossible to target the eradication of poverty without impacting on child and adolescent mental health. Although out of the realm of the health sector, the activities for poverty eradication, such as policies of gender equality, legal protection, economic opportunities, improved schooling and housing, promote child and adolescent mental health (Omigbodun, 2011).[25]

Poverty's most devastating effects are on children, to whom it poses a great threat. It affects their

> *education, health, nutrition, and security. It also negatively affects the emotional and spiritual development of children through the environment it creates(SDGs).*

Goal 2:   Zero Hunger

This goal has specific targets to enable infants' access to safe, nutritious and sufficient food all year round, which will help to reduce the incidence of intellectual disability and enhance cognitive performance of infants, children and adolescents.

Goal 3:   Good Health and Well-being

Ensure healthy lives and promote well-being for all at all ages.

Goal 3 has strong targets for mental health, which include prevention and treatment of mental disorders, and promotion of mental health and well-being, as well as tackling of substance abuse.

> *By 2030, reduce by one-third premature mortality from non-communicable diseases through prevention and treatment, and promote mental health and well-being. Strengthen the prevention and treatment of substance abuse, including narcotic drug abuse and harmful use of alcohol.*

Goal 4:   Quality Education

Ensure inclusive and equitable quality education and promote lifelong learning opportunities for all

Goal 4 looks at mental health promoting educational activities and stresses quality early childhood development and supportive learning environ-ments for children.

Goal 5:   Gender Equality

Achieve gender equality and empower all women and girls

Goal 5 tackles discrimination against girls and encourages protection from harmful practices that damage mental health such as child marriage, violence, sexual exploitation and female genital mutilation.

Goal 8:   Decent Work and Economic Growth

> *By 2030, achieve full and productive employment and decent work for all women and men, including for young people and persons with disabilities, immediate and effective measures to eradicate forced labour, end modern slavery and human trafficking and secure the prohibition and elimination of the worst forms of child labour, including recruitment and use of child soldiers, and by 2025, end child labour in all its forms.*

Goal 16:   Peace, Justice and Strong Institutions

> *Promote peaceful and inclusive societies for sustainable development, provide access to justice for all and build effective, accountable and inclusive institutions at all levels.*

This focuses on ending abuse, exploitation, trafficking and all forms of violence against and torture of children. It also has targets to substantially reduce corruption and bribery in all its forms.

The UN in a recent report[5] stressed the belief that the energies of the large and increasing youthful population in sub-Saharan Africa can be channelled along the path of economic and social growth. The premise on which this is built is that the "economic miracle" experienced by East Asia can be a reality in SSA if care is taken to ensure that the mental health of children and adolescents is promoted.

The goals and targets of the SDGs overlap greatly with the United Nations Convention on the Rights of the Child. The Convention on Rights of the Child [35] is a human rights treaty which is a formally concluded and a ratified agreement between states. As at now, 195 countries have ratified it, the major exceptions being the United States and South Sudan. Out of the 41 articles in Part 1 of the Rights of the Child, 25 (Over 60%) have direct implications for the development of mental health services, research and training for CAMH care within countries. Table 2 below reveals that there are rights to promote mental health, prevent or protect from mental illness, treat mental illness and rehabilitate children with mental disabilities. These are also in synergy with the SDGs.

Table 2. Mental health rights in the Convention of the Rights of the Child

Article	Mental Health Promotion 'Rights'
3	Safe, healthy institutions with adequate and suitable staff
7	Cared for by parents
12	Be heard
13	Freedom of expression
14	Freedom of thought
17	Access to resources aimed at promoting mental health
18	Mentally healthy environments
27	Standard of living adequate for mental...development
28	Primary education, compulsory, available & free to all
29	Development of child's mental abilities to fullest potential
31	Rest and leisure

Article	Mental Ill-Health Prevention 'Rights'
9	Not separated from parents except in cases of abuse/neglect
19	Protect from all forms of physical or mental violence, injury or abuse/neglect
32	Protect from hazardous work harmful to health or physical or mental development
33	Protect from illicit use and trafficking of narcotic drugs & psychotropic substances
34	Protect from all forms of sexual exploitation and abuse
35	Prevent abduction, sale or traffic in children
36	Protect against all other forms of exploitation
37	Protect from torture, inhumane treatment or punishment
38	Do not take a direct part in hostilities
Article	**Mental Ill-Health Treatment 'Rights'**
24	Enjoy the highest attainable standard of health and facilities for the treatment of illness and rehabilitation of health.
25	Receive treatment for a physical or mental health disorder, to a periodic review of the treatment and all other circumstances relevant to the placement
Article	**Mental Disability Rehabilitation 'Rights'**
23	Children with mental and physical disabilities should enjoy a full and decent life in conditions which ensure dignity, self-reliance and facilitate active participation
39	Appropriate measures to promote physical and psychological recovery, and social reintegration of victims of neglect, exploitation, abuse, torture or armed conflicts
40	Those who commit crimes should be treated in a manner consistent with the promotion of the child's sense of dignity and worth
40	Facilities for counselling; probation; foster care; education and vocational training programmes among other alternatives to institutional care shall be available

In a letter dated December 16, 2010, the John D. and Catherine T. MacArthur Foundation informed the Vice Chancellor of the University of Ibadan that a grant had been approved for building Child and Adolescent Mental Health (CAMH) capacity in sub-Saharan Africa through the university. This was to be executed primarily through the development and implementation of a master of science degree programme in child and adolescent mental health (MSc. CAMH).

Once training activities commenced in January 2013, the course leaders, tutors and administrative team in CCAMH have sustained momentum and in a record time of four and a half (4½) years trained 60 CAMH professionals from 8 countries in sub-Saharan Africa. Eritrea, Ghana, Liberia, Kenya, Nigeria, Sierra Leone, Zambia and Zimbabwe now have at least one fully trained professional to lead service development, teach and conduct research in CAMH. The impact of CCAMH can be seen in the areas of training, research and service.

Prior to the establishment of CCAMH, there was no formal training of CAMH professionals in sub-Saharan Africa with the exception of South Africa, and there were very few services to cater to the identified burden of mental health problems in the region's largely youthful population.

CCAMH is now filling up the void with regular and coordinated training, research and provision of services for evidence-based CAMH care. Implementing the multidisciplinary leadership training programme in CCAMH is also directed at increasing the probability of professionals remaining in the region to carry out CAMH care.

CCAMH is also changing the landscape of research in sub-Saharan Africa. In an editorial to introduce the research work of CCAMH's students, Omigbodun and Belfer stressed that the wide disparity in scientific research on CAMH originates from low resource settings like SSA when compared to high resource settings.[11] In addition to the gap, the virtual absence of CAMH research and publications hindered CAMH's policy development as well as the advocacy drive for service development and training programmes.

With this sustained research output from CCAMH, the means to provide for advocacy are gradually being put in place and the trained CAMH professionals can utilize available tools to make a difference. So far, 10 students have published their works with all students as being first and corresponding authors as can be seen from the list below:

Publications from the MSc. CAMH research projects so far

1. **Abdulmalik J**, Ani C, Ajuwon A, Omigbodun O. (2016).[36] Effects of problem-solving interventions on aggressive behaviours among primary school pupils in Ibadan, Nigeria. *Journal of Child and Adolescent Psychiatry and Mental Health* http://www.biomedcentral.com/c ollections/child-psychiatry-in -africa

2. **Abubakar-Abdullateef A**, Adedokun B, Omigbodun O. (2017).[32] A comparative study of the prevalence and correlates of psychiatric disorders in Almajiris and public primary school pupils in Zaria, northwest Nigeria. *Journal of Child and Adolescent Psychiatry and Mental Health* 11. doi:10.1186/s13034-017-0166-3

3. **Adeniyi YC**, Omigbodun OO. (2016).[37] Effect of a classroom-based intervention on the social skills of pupils with intellectual disability in southwest Nigeria. *Journal of Child and Adolescent Psychiatry and Mental Health* http://www.biomedcentral.com/collections/child-psychiatry-in -africa

4. **Bella-Awusah T,** Ani C, Ajuwon A, Omigbodun O. (2016).[38] Effectiveness of brief school-based, group cognitive behavioural therapy for depressed adolescents in southwest Nigeria. *Journal of Child and Adolescent Psychiatry and Mental Health* http://www.onlinelibrary@wiley.com/doi/10.1111/camh.12104/a bstract

5. **Bello-Mojeed MA.,** Ani C, Lagunju I, Omigbodun O. (2016).[39] The effect of parent-mediated behavioural interventionfor aggression in children with autism spectrum disorder in Lagos Nigeria. *Journal of Child and Adolescent Psychiatry and Mental Health* http://www.biomedcentral.com/c ollections/child-psychiatry-in - africa

6. **Ekore RI.,** Ajuwon AJ, Abdulmalik JO, Omigbodun OO, Bella-Awusah TT. (2016).[40] Developing mental health peer counselling services for undergraduate students of a Nigerian university: A pilot study. *Ife PsychologIA 2016, 24(2), 246-258 http:www.questia.com/library/ournal/1P3-4317230631/developing-mental-peer-counselling-services*

7. **Kamau J,** Omigbodun O, Bella-Awusah T, Adedokun B. (2017).[41] Who seeks child and adolescent mental healthcare in Kenya? A descriptive clinic profile at a tertiary referral facility. *JournalofChildandAdolescent Psychiatry and Mental Health www.ncbi.nlm.nih.gov/pubmed/28293286*

8. **Lasisi D,** Ani C, Lasebikan V, Sheik L, Omigbodun O. (2017).[42] Effect of attention deficithyperactivity disorder training programme on the knowledge and attitudes of primary school teachers in Kaduna, northwest Nigeria. *Journal of Child* and Adolescent Psychiatry and Mental http://rdcu.be/qfQL

9. **Oduguwa A,** Adedokun B, Omigbodun O. (2017).[43] Effect of a mental health training programme on Nigerian school pupils' perception of mental illness. *Journal of Child and Adolescent Psychiatry and Mental Health* https://capmh.biomedcentral.com/articles/10.1186/s13034-017-0157-4

10. **Okewole A,** Adewuya AO, Bella-Awusah T, Ani C, Ajuwon A, Omigbodun O. (2016).[44] Maternal Depression and Child psychopathology among attendees at a child neuropsychiatric clinic in Abeokuta, Nigeria: A cross sectional study. *Journal of Child and Adolescent Psychiatry and Mental Health* http://www.biomedcentral.com/c ollections/child-psychiatry-in - africa

Conclusion

The mental health of children and adolescents in sub Saharan Africa is the foundation for the wealth of this region. With a decline in child mortality, social and health interventions need to move towards creating a mental health promoting environment for the youth who will remain alive and form the future. The whole community must get involved in instituting measures that will promote the mental well-being of children and adolescents while preventing mental disorders, treating those who have mental disorders and providing for their rehabilitation. The picture of CAMH in sub-Saharan Africa used to be bleak, but now changing through concerted efforts. A great deal of work is being done to lay a firm foundation for the building of capacity for child and adolescent mental health in sub-Saharan Africa. Child and adolescent mental health is at the centre of the health of the community because children are the future of any society, for *there is no child and adolescent health without child and adolescent mental health.*

Learning points & objectives

- Define Child and Adolescent Mental Health (CAMH)
- Describe CAMH Protective and Risk Factors in the Family, School and Community
- Outline the History of CAMH in sub-Saharan Africa (SSA)
- Describe Results of Epidemiological Studies on CAMH in SSA
- Describe Available Tools to Drive the CAMH Agenda in SSA

References

1. WHO. Mental Health Action Plan 2013-2020. World Health Organization, Geneva, 2013.
2. WHO, World Psychiatric Association and International Association of Child and Adolescent Psychiatry and Allied Professions. *Atlas: Child and Adolescent Mental Health Resources: Global Concerns, Implications for the Future*, World Health Organization, Geneva, 2005.
3. WHO. *Child and Adolescent Mental Health Policies and Plans*, Geneva, World Health Organization, Geneva, 2005.
4. Sameroff AJ, Seifer R, Barocas R, Zax M, Greenspan S. Intelligence quotient scores of 4-year-old children: Social-environmental risk factors. *Pediatrics* 1987; 79: 343-350.
5. United Nations. Millennium development goals. http://www.un.org/millennium goals/(Accessed on 23 August 2011).
6. Omigbodun OO, Bella TT. Obstetric risk factors and subsequent mental health problems in a child psychiatry clinic population in Nigeria. *Tropical Journal of Obstetrics and Gynaecology* 2004; 21: 15-20.
7. Graham P, Orley J. WHO and the mental health of children. *World Health Forum* 1998; 19(3):268-72.
8. Olatawura M. Mental health services for children in the African region. *International Journal of Mental Health* 1978; 7: 34-38.
9. Robertson B, Omigbodun O, Gaddour N. Child and adolescent psychiatry in Africa: Luxury or necessity? Guest editorial. *African Journal of Psychiatry* 2010; 13: 329-331.
10. Garralda EM, Raynaud J. *Increasing Awareness of Child and Adolescent Mental Health*. International Association for Child and Adolescent Psychiatry and Allied Profession, Paris, 2010.
11. Omigbodun OO, Belfer ML.. Building research capacity for child and adolescent mental health in Africa. *Child and Adolescent Psychiatry and Mental Health* 2016; 10: 27.
12. UNICEF. Statistics and Monitoring, 2008. www.unicef.org/statistics/ (Accessed on 19 June 2017).
13. Kieling C, Baker-Henningham H, Belfer M, Conti G, Ertem I, Omigbodun O, Rohde La, Srinath S, Ulkuer N, Rahman A. 2011. Child and adolescent mental health worldwide: Evidence for action. *The Lancet* 2011; 378: 1515-1525.

14. Jegede O, Cederblad M. Problemes de saute mentale des enfants du Nigeria. *Livre Annual de L'Association Internationale de Psychiatrie de L'Enfant et de L'adolescent et des Professions Associees. L'Enfant dans sa Famille,* 1990; 9: 519-528.

15. Maulik PK, Mascarenhas MN, Mathers CD, Dua T, Saxena S. Prevalence of intellectual disability: A meta-analysis of population-based studies. *Research in Developmental Disabilities* 2011; 32: 419-436.

16. Adewuya AO, Famuyiwa OO. Attention deficit hyperactivity disorder among Nigerian primary school children: Prevalence and co-morbid conditions. *European Child & Adolescent Psychiatry* 2007; 16: 10-15.

17. Alikor EAD, Frank-briggs AI, Okoh BAN. Attention deficit hyperactivity disorder among school children in Port Harcourt, Nigeria. *American Journal of Psychiatry and Neuroscience* 2015; 3(2): 23-29.

18. Ashenafi Y, Kebede D, Desta M, Alem A. Prevalence of mental and behavioural disorders in Ethiopian children. *East Afr Med J,* 2001; 78: 308-311.

19. Fatiregun AA, Kumapayi TE. Prevalence and correlates of depressive symptoms among in-school adolescents in a rural district in southwest Nigeria. *J Adolesc,* 2014; 37: 197-203.

20. Donnir G, Kusi-Mensah K, Owusu-Antwi R, Wemakor S, Omigbodun O. Prevalence and Pattern of Mental Disorders in Primary School Children and Correlates with Academic Achievment in Kumasi, Ghana. *The 22nd International Association for Child and Adolescent Psychiatry and Allied Professions World Congress.* Calgary, Canada, 2016.

21. Ndetei DM, Mutiso V, Musyimi C, Mokaya AG, Anderson KK, Mckenzie K, Musau A. 2016. The prevalence of mental disorders among upper primary school children in Kenya. *Soc Psychiatry Psychiatr Epidemiol* 2016; 51: 63-71.

22. Abbo C, Kinyanda E, Kizza RB, Levin J, Ndyanabangi S, Stein DJ. Prevalence, comorbidity and predictors of anxiety disorders in children and adolescents in rural north-eastern Uganda. *Child Adolesc Psychiatry Ment Health,* 2013; 7: 21.

23. Omigbodun O, Dogra N, Esan O, Adedokun B. Prevalence and correlates of suicidal behaviour among adolescents in southwest Nigeria. *International Journal of Social Psychiatry* 2008; 54: 34-46.

24. Omigbodun OO. A cost-effective model for increasing access to

mental health care at the primary care level in Nigeria. *Journal of Mental Health Policy and Economics* 2001; 4: 133-140.

25. Omigbodun OO. Unifying Psyche and Soma for Child Healthcare in Nigeria The 35th Annual General and Scientfic Meeting of the West African College of Physicians (WACP), Nigerian Chapter, Lagos, 2011.

26. Ibeziako P, Bella T, Omigbodun O, Belfer M. Teachers' perspectives of mental health needs in Nigerian schools. *Journal of Child & Adolescent Mental Health,* 2009; 21: 147-156.

27. CRCPC. CRC Adoption, Signatures and Ratification. CRC Policy Centre, Cyprus.

28. Brides GN. 2015. Child marriage in sub Saharan Africa. Ending child marriage in Africa. http://www.girlsnotbrides.org/about-girls-not-brides (Accessed on 14th July 2017).

29. Abiodun O. Emotional illness in a paediatric population in Nigeria. *East African Medical Journal* 1992; 69: 557-559.

30. Olley B. Social and health behaviors in youth of the streets of Ibadan, Nigeria. *Child Abuse & Neglect* 2006; 30: 271-282.

31. Abdulmalik J, Omigbodun O, Beida O, Adedokun B. Psychoactive substance use among children in informal religious schools (Almajiris) in northern Nigeria. *Mental Health, Religion and Culture* 2009; 12: 527-542.

32. Abubakar-Abdullateef A, Adedokun B, Omigbodun O. A comparative study of the prevalence and correlates of psychiatric disorders in Almajiris and public primary school pupils in Zaria, Northwest Nigeria. *Child and Adolescent Psychiatry and Mental Health* 2017; 11: 29.

33. Omigbodun OO. Psychosocial issues in a child and adolescent psychiatric clinic population in Nigeria. *Social Psychiatry and Psychiatric Epidemiology* 2004; 39: 667-672.

34. UNDP. Sustainable Development Goals. http://www.undp.org/content/undp/en/home/sustainable-development-goals.html [Accessed on 14th July 2017).

35. UN. United Nations Treaty Collection . United Nations, New York, 1990.

36. Abdulmalik J, Ani C, Ajuwon AJ, Omigbodun O. Effects of problem-solving interventions on aggressive behaviours among primary school pupils in Ibadan, Nigeria. *Child and Adolescent Psychiatry and Mental Health* 2016; 10: 31.

37. Adeniyi YC, Omigbodun OO. Effect of a classroom-based intervention on the social skills of pupils with intellectual disability in Southwest Nigeria. *Child and Adolescent Psychiatry and Mental Health* 2016; 10, 29.

38. Bella Awusah T, Ani C, Ajuwon A, Omigbodun O. 2016. Effectiveness of brief school based, group cognitive behavioural therapy for depressed adolescents in southwest Nigeria. *Child and Adolescent Psychiatry and Mental Health* 2016; 21: 44-50.

39. Bello-Mojeed M, Ani C, Lagunju I, Omigbodun O. Feasibility of parent-mediated behavioural intervention for behavioural problems in children with Autism Spectrum Disorder in Nigeria: a pilot study. *Child and Adolescent Psychiatry and Mental Health* 2016: 10:, 28.

40. Ekore R, Ajuwon A, Abdulmalik J, Bella-Awusah T. Developing mental health peer counselling services for undergraduate students of a Nigerian University: A pilot study. *IFE PsychologIA: An International Journal* 2016; 24: 246-258.

41. Kamau JW, Omigbodun OO, Bella-Awusah T, Adedokun B. Who seeks child and adolescent mental health care in Kenya? A descriptive clinic profile at a tertiary referral facility. *Child and Adolescent Psychiatry and Mental Health* 2017; 11: 14.

42. Lasisi D, Ani C, Lasebikan V, Sheikh L, Omigbodun O. Effect of attention-deficit–hyperactivity-disorder training program on the knowledge and attitudes of primary school teachers in Kaduna, North West Nigeria. *Child and Adolescent Psychiatry and Mental Health* 2017; 11:, 15.

43. Oduguwa AO, Adedokun B, Omigbodun OO. Effect of a mental health training programme on Nigerian school pupils' perceptions of mental illness. *Child and Adolescent Psychiatry and Mental Health* 2017; 11: 19.

44. Okewole AO, Adewuya AO, Ajuwon AJ, Bella-Awusah TT, Omigbodun OO. Maternal depression and child psychopathology among attendees at a Child Neuropsychiatric Clinic in Abeokuta, Nigeria: a cross sectional study. *Child and Adolescent Psychiatry and Mental Health* 2016; 10: 30.

7

Intellectual Disability (Learning Disability)

Yetunde C. Adeniyi, Taiwo Adewumi

Definition of intellectual disability

Intellectual disability (ID) or mental retardation is defined as

> . . . a condition of arrested or incomplete development of the mind, which is especially characterized by impairment of skills manifested during the developmental period, which contribute to the overall level of intelligence, i.e., cognitive, language, motor, and social abilities.[1]

The American Association on Intellectual and Developmental Disabilities (AAIDD) defines it as "limitations both in intellectual functioning and adaptive behaviour."[2] Harris reported the prevalence of ID to vary between 1% and 3% globally.[3] The health condition currently being referred to as "intellectual disability" (ID) is a cluster of syndromes and disorders characterized by low intelligence and associated limitations in adaptive behaviour.[4,1] The disorder is evident before 18 years of age and occurs on a continuum from mild to profound intellectual disability.[1]

Prevalence and diagnostic criteria

The overall prevalence of ID is about 1% - 3% worldwide[5] but it varies across countries. The prevalence is around 1% in high income countries and 2% -3% in low and middle income (LAMI) countries.[6,7] Aetiological factors such as malnutrition, lack of perinatal care, and exposure to toxic and infectious agents, which are more common in (LAMI) countries[8] may contribute to higher prevalence rates of intellectual disability reported in the LAMI countries.[9,10,8] The prevalence is slightly higher in boys, which is explained by hereditary factors, such as X-linked intellectual disability[11] and biological characteristics of brain development which supports higher levels of developmental disorders in boys.[12]

The American Psychiatric Association's (APA) diagnostic criteria for intellectual disability (ID, formerly mental retardation) is found in the Diagnostic and Statistical Manual of Mental Disorders (DSM-5).[13] A summary of the diagnostic criteria in DSM-5 is as follows.

1. Deficits in intellectual functioning[13]

This includes various mental abilities such as: reasoning, problem solving, planning, abstract thinking, judgment, academic learning (ability to learn in school via traditional teaching methods), experiential learning (the ability to learn through experience, trial and error, and observation). These mental abilities are measured using the IQ tests. A score of approximately two standard deviations below average represents a significant cognitive deficit; this is typically an IQ score of 70 or below.[13]

On the whole, intelligence refers to a general mental capacity. It involves the ability to reason, plan, solve problems, think abstractly, comprehend complex ideas, learn quickly and learn from experience. It is often represented by Intelligent Quotient (IQ) Scores. Cognition on the other hand is the broad term used to designate all the processes involved in "knowing" such as perception, attention, thinking, memory, intelligence and language.

Measurement of intelligence is usually a reference to a quantitative assessment of sub groups, or combination of sub groups of cognitive abilities as the scores of which are most commonly combined and quantified in Intelligent Quotient. The intelligence quotient for the normal population falls between IQ: 80-120. IQ < 70 is considered as intellectual disability. The severity of intellectual impairment can be further categorised based on the IQ scores from the least to the most affected as follows:

- IQ 70-79 Borderline
- IQ 50-69 Mild (85% of people with ID)
- IQ 35-49 Moderate (10% of people with ID)
- IQ 20-34 Severe (3-4% of people with ID)
- IQ< 20 Profound (1-2% of people with ID)

2. Deficits or impairments in adaptive functioning[13]

This includes the skills needed to live in an independent and responsible manner. Limited abilities in these life skills make it difficult to achieve age-appropriate standards of behaviour.

Without these skills, a person needs additional support to succeed at school, work, or independent life.[14]

Adaptive behaviour is a developmental and social construct that describes the fundamental ways an individual typically responds to various situations; it is dependent upon both developmental status and cultural expectations. The measurement of adaptive behaviour assesses performance in school, the ability to care for oneself at home, and in interaction with peers and adults, and level of independence in a variety of settings. It includes two basic concepts

(1) age-appropriate self-sufficiency (carrying out of activities of daily living) and

(2) social competence

Deficits in adaptive functioning are measured using standardized, culturally appropriate tests. These skills include:

i. **Communication skills:** This refers to the ability to convey information from one person to another. This information is communicated through words and actions. It involves the ability to understand others, and to express one's self through words or actions.

ii. **Social skills:** This refers to the ability to interact effectively with others. Social skills are critical for success in life. These skills include the ability to understand and comply with social rules, customs, and standards of public behaviour. This intricate function requires the ability to process figurative language and detect unspoken cues such as body language.

iii. **Personal independence at home or in community settings:** This refers to the ability to take care of oneself. Some examples are bathing, dressing, and feeding. It also includes the ability to safely complete day-to-day tasks without guidance.[14] Some examples of these tasks are cooking, cleaning, and laundry. There are also routine activities performed in the community. This includes shopping, and accessing public transportation and other services.

iv. **School or work functioning:** This refers to the ability to conform to the social standards at work or school. It includes the ability to learn new knowledge, skills, and abilities.

3. These limitations occur during the developmental period

This means problems with intellectual and/or adaptive functioning are evident during childhood or adolescence, usually before 18 years. This thus differentiates them from adult-onset cognitive or adaptive regressions.

Causes of ID with emphasis on sub-Saharan Africa

Prenatal, peri-natal and post natal influences can cause intellectual disability during this delicate period. Some perinatal causes that can affect the baby include alcohol and substance abuse by the pregnant mother, bleeding during pregnancy and illness or injury of the mother during pregnancy. Recent research has implicated smoking as an increased risk for prematurity[9] and this can lead to intellectual disability. Extreme prematurity, low birth weight and brain injury[10,9] are common perinatal causes. Postnatal illnesses which can result in intellectual disability are meningitis, encephalitis, measles, pertussis (whooping cough), head injuries and other traumas to young children.[8] Genetic or inherited causes include Down syndrome, which is the most common genetic condition associated with intellectual disability, and Fragile X syndrome which is the most common identifiable inherited cause of intellectual disability.

Environmental causes include cultural deprivation and extreme poverty, which can result in malnutrition, inadequate medical care or environmental hazards.[8] Developing regions such as Nigeria tend to have abundance of environmental hazards. Many of the other environmental factors especially toxins have not been adequately investigated in the LAMI countries, hence there is limited evidence about the contributions of environmental toxins and hazards to the development of ID in LAMI countries.

Nomenclature issues around ID

At the end of the 19th century, Down (1887) proposed a medical paradigm of disability, in series of lectures titled: *Some of the mental afflictions of childhood and youth*. In that context, he proposed changes in the terminologies of disability and a scientific classification to define it. He also suggested that terminologies such as, "idiot" and "imbecile" were inappropriate and should be replaced with "moron" and "feebleminded.".

Several names have been used to describe the entity currently called intellectual disability; names like backward, feebleminded, idiot, imbecile, moron, mental handicap and mental retardation.[15] Currently, intellectual disability is an established diagnosis in the different psychiatric diagnostic tools, including the International classification of Diseases[1] and the Diagnostic Statistical Manual of Mental Disorders.[13] Despite the fact that many parts of the world have been able to successfully transit this change in nomenclature, most parts of Africa have not been very successful due to inadequate training and poorly coordinated programmes. For example in a need assessment done at a special school in Nigeria, it was found out that the teachers still use some of the out-dated terminologies as well as criteria to place children in classes, these terms include 'educable', 'trainable' and 'profound or 'untrainable' mentally retarded.[16]

Although these designations appear to provide ease of grouping to the teachers and help them to draw boundaries between individual students or groups, they, however, have the tendency to exclude children who are grouped as untrainable–not able to benefit from available services. It can also affect their eligibility or ineligibility to be part of a service, or whether they are included or not included in a benefit such as protection against discrimination. These limitations could be more marked in settings where resources are scarce, such as in the LAMI countries.

Co-morbid mental disorders and diagnostic over-shadowing: impact on physical health and morbidity

For many years, professionals and researchers did not believe that intellectual disability and mental illness could both be present in the same person, as a result, this was not studied.

Most of the research on this topic has occurred in the last few decades. These studies have shown that the full range of mental disorders that are present in persons with intellectual disability[17] and at rates that are four to five times higher than what is seen in the general population.[18] Some studies show that about 30-60% of persons with ID have a diagnosable mental disorder.[19,17,5] In particular, common co-morbid conditions are autism, self-injurious behaviour, attention deficit hyperactivity disorder, anxiety, depression and psychosis.[5]

Mental health problems also occur in people with ID just like in the general population, but can be hard to diagnose. Intellectual disability likely contributes to the diagnostic overshadowing bias, which describes the tendency of the clinicians to overlook other symptoms of mental health problems in persons with ID. People with intellectual disabilities (ID) are particularly vulnerable to health problems and experience difficulties in meeting their healthcare needs.[20,21] The prevalence of mental health problems among people with ID varies in different studies (from 14% to 60%) and can be difficult to identify and diagnose.[22] Another reason for this difficulty is the considerable overlap between mental health problems and the challenging behaviours of persons with intellectual disability.

The higher rate of mental health problems among children with ID should be of concern because these problems can have a negative effect on the well-being, social inclusion and life opportunities of these children.[23] Moreover, mental health problems in this population can lead to residential placement and can have a negative impact on the well-being of their families.[23]

There are several modalities for preventing and treating co-morbid mental health problems in children and adolescents with ID. Sarimiski suggested that early interventions may help to prevent emotional and behavioural problems among them. This can be achieved by encouraging a positive parent-child relationship, increasing the parents' educational competence as well as understanding of ID and how it impacts the child's functioning, supporting the children to develop positive relationships with their peers, and promoting their social skills and competence.[24]

Intellectual disability is also associated with a wide range of medical conditions that have diverse effects on the physical health of the individual.[21] Studies have shown that certain health conditions are more prevalent among the ID population.[25] Some of the more common health conditions among people with ID include motor deficits, epilepsy, allergies, otitis media, gastroesophageal reflux disease (GERD), dysmenorrhea, sleep disturbances, visual and hearing impairments, oral health problems, and constipation.[26,25]

Many times, the health problems of people with ID often go undiagnosed and untreated, due to difficulties with communication.[27] Undiagnosed and untreated health problems may reduce a person's life expectancy and contribute to the development of secondary health complications.[27,28]

Table 1 The prevalence of mental health problems among children and adolescents with and without intellectual disabilities

Psychiatric Disorder	With ID (%)	Without ID (%)
Any Psychiatric Disorder	36	8
Any Emotional Disorder	12	4
Separation Anxiety	3	0.7
Generalised Anxiety Disorder	2	<1
Tic Disorders	<1	<1 (x5)
Any Conduct Disorder	21	4
Oppositional Defiant Disorder	11	2
Hyperactivity Disorder	8	1
ASD	8	1
Eating Disorders	0.4	0.1
1 Psychiatric Disorder	19	6
2 Psychiatric Disorders	16	2
> 2 Psychiatric Disorders	3	1

Source: The mental health of children and adolescents with learning disabilities in Britain. Institute of health Research, Lancaster University[29]

The following factors have been found to contribute to the higher prevalence of mental health problems in persons with intellectual disability:

- Poor communication
- Sensory disability

- Epilepsy
- Physical illness
- Limited range of coping strategies
- Medication
- Social factors – abuse and neglect, schooling issues, poverty, parental psychiatric disorder, transgenerational social disadvantage, bereavement, life events, daily hassles, post-traumatic stress disorder, migration, attachment disorders
- Behavioural phenotypes
- Severity of the learning disability
- Cause of the learning disability
- Presence of ASD

Mental health assessment and treatment

The same principles and practice of assessment and treatment of mental health disorders apply to people with ID as with non-ID populations. A holistic approach using the bio-psycho-social model is a helpful framework. It is imperative to rule out any organic causes and avoid diagnostic overshadowing and ensure that physical health issues are treated adequately and timely.

Important points to consider

i. **What are you being asked to assess:** Children with ID are often referred for varying types of assessment. Sometimes the referral and request for assessment might be specific such as assessing for co-morbid psychiatric, behavioural or a physical disorder. Sometimes this could be a part of risk assessment for placement, capacity or consent issues.

ii. **Where are you going to get information from:** Can patient communicate verbally or use other communication aids, speaking to carers and significant others which include educating staff and other professionals involved. It is important to consider the patient's developmental level and not just the chronological age in interpreting the presentation as behaviour may be appropriate for the developmental level. If there is no verbal communication, there is still a wealth of information that can be obtained through:

- Observation
- Appearance: signs of neglect, level of self-care, mobility, physical disability, nutritional status
- Behaviour: Stereotypic behaviour, self-injurious behaviour sometimes evidenced by scars around the wrist and back of hands, tics, possible seizures
- Communication: verbal communication, gestures, signing
- Mood: smiling, wailing, crying, biological features of depression and mania
- Perceptions: perplexity, response to abnormal stimuli

What is the individual's usual level of functioning?

- Previous IQ assessment, e.g., WISC, WAIS, if any
- Type of schooling: Mainstream, special or inclusive type.
- Daily living skills including communication, ability to form relationships, toileting skills, feeding strengths.
- Rituals, obsessions, tics and seizures should be observed.

All treatment options appropriate to non-ID population should be considered. These include pharmacological and non-pharmacological options.

Non-pharmacological treatment may include behavioural treatments such as applied behavioural analysis (ABA), positive reinforcement. Other psychological interventions, e.g., cognitive behaviour therapy (CBT) can be adapted and used successfully in patients with ID.

In pharmacological interventions, be mindful of the overuse of sedatives and tranquilizers and the need to closely monitor both therapeutic and adverse effects. The rule in the use of medication in ID is to 'start low and go slow'; doses should be titrated more slowly due to increased risk of side effects and the minimum effective dose should be used. Other factors to consider include:

- Note that antipsychotics are epileptogenic; therefore, caution should be exercised in their use in individuals with epilepsy
- Target and treat symptoms and test medication

- Obtain consent from the person if possible, or agreement from carers before commencing treatment
- Do not let fear of capacity and consent issues prevent the patient from having appropriate medical care
- Maintain the dignity of the patient at all times

Life expectancy of individuals with ID

Generally, when compared to the general population, persons with an intellectual disability have lower life expectancy, higher morbidity, higher rates of unmet health needs, and more difficulty in finding and getting health care. This is worse among those with severe and profound forms of ID and those living in institutions.[30]

Although the life expectancy of people with ID is increasing, it still remains lower than that of the general population. It seems that ageing starts earlier in persons with ID. Advances in medicine, health care, nutrition and community inclusion have resulted in more children with ID living on to adulthood.

Recent surveys have reported that the life expectancy of people with ID has increased significantly during the past few decades from about a mean age at death of 19 years in the 1930s to about 66 years in1990s; adults with ID are living longer. It has also been suggested that many persons with ID will live as long as the general population. This significant increase has left the problem of transition from paediatric and youth services to adult health care services.[31]

Teaching ID in medical curriculum and curriculum for training teachers

Exposure to intellectual disability training in the undergraduate curriculum is limited and teaching on this topic appears fragmented and inadequate. A proper curriculum should not only aim to teach knowledge but should provide skills and teach on attitude towards individuals with ID and their families. Piachaud[32] suggested that teaching strategies such as visiting clinics and services, interviewing and assessing patients with disabilities under supervision all provide direct opportunities for the three areas of learning. Other suggested strategies include formal teaching, video material and a series of home visits. Meeting a family, understanding the difficulties faced by parents, and learning to listen and demonstrate interested concern are important goals. The teaching of the knowledge of ID should include facts and figures, aetiology, epidemiology and the concepts of disability.

Skills in communication, examination, assessment and diagnosis of people with learning disability can be learned in existing clinic or community settings. The integration of disability and rehabilitation should be incorporated into clinical teaching, with the focus of teaching on those types of disability which are common in the community. There should be a greater emphasis on functional assessment when teaching physical examination, and a wider use of standard assessment instruments, for example, what activities of daily living can ID patient perform, level of cognitive ability and locomotor disability.

Some requirements for effective inclusion of ID teaching in medical students' curricula include a well-coordinated programme, including an agreed set of training objectives throughout medical school; trained personnel; and proper coordination among the specialties of medicine that are involved. The specialist in the psychiatry of learning disability is well placed to be the coordinator of learning disability teaching in medical school, although others may also contribute to that role. It is good to start with a definition of what is to be taught in each department and who takes responsibility for the teaching. Other departments that should be included are: public health, paediatrics, general practice and neurology.

Educational provisions and support for people with ID: inclusive education/specialist provision

Children and adolescents with intellectual disabilities are a very heterogeneous group[33], making it difficult to design a general school curriculum for them. For example, children and adolescents with profound intellectual disability will need their education to focus on training in self-care skills such as feeding, dressing, and toileting. Children with moderate intellectual disability who have some self-care skills may study to obtain skills for employment, transportation, recreation, cooking, and other social skills. Children with mild intellectual disabilities can function in basic academic courses.[33]

Two important issues have dominated the educational policies and practices for students with intellectual disabilities in the last few years in developed settings. The first aspect is what should be taught to such students and who should teach them, and the second issue is where they should be taught—in 'inclusive' settings alongside normal peers or in special settings dedicated to their needs.[33]

The current trend in the education of children and adolescents with intellectual disability is to remove them from institutions and put them in inclusive settings.[34,8] This process of de-institutionalization for intellectual disability services is at different stages across the world; while there is complete closure in Sweden, most countries in Asia and Africa are still educating persons with ID separately in institutions and special schools.[35,36]

Some of the barriers to inclusive education of children with intellectual disabilities include the fact that parents are reluctant to send their children and adolescents with disabilities to regular schools that are of poor quality and not welcoming to their children.[37] Another barrier is that parents may not see the value of sending a child and adolescent with ID to school because they may not see this as a good investment.[37] Another important obstacle is that regular teachers are not adequately trained to teach children with ID in assertive and social skills.[38]

In addition, there are very few training centres for special needs teachers, and sadly, the few special needs teachers often end up in mainstream schools in the private sector due to better remuneration. Currently, there are no structured educational plans and packages for this population in most parts of sub-Saharan Africa. For instance, in Nigeria, teachers in schools for persons with intellectual disability are provided with the same curriculum as for mainstream schools. The mainstream school curriculum caters for core academic content areas like writing, reading and mathematics and fails to address issues such as adaptive functioning.[16]

Multidisciplinary approach to the care of persons with ID

A multi-disciplinary team is used to describe a group of professionals from different disciplines who meet on a regular basis to share information and plan services in a co-ordinated manner. Ongoing de-institutionalization has resulted in several problems in medical care delivery to people with intellectual disability, such as an increased workload for general practitioners (GPs) and a lack of active co-ordination and co-operation between healthcare professionals. A major consequence is the incidence of untreated yet treatable medical conditions.

An integrated care approach may provide a means for better co-ordination and delivery of care. Even though the potential advantages of integrated care are well known, the applicability of this approach for people with intellectual disability is still to be demonstrated especially in low and middle-income countries.

In Nigeria, this is mainly as a result of inadequate professionals and the uneven distribution of the few available ones between the major cities and other parts of the country. Other reasons are rural-urban migration, professional brain drain due to political and economic instability. The team members should include:

- Child psychiatrist
- Occupational therapist
- Nurse
- Paediatrician
- Physiotherapist
- Psychologist
- Special education teacher
- Speech and language therapist (SALT)
- Social worker

Community inclusion and other services for persons with ID in Nigeria, compared with best practice

There is now a shift towards moving people out of institutions and into the community and with this shift, it is necessary to ensure that there are appropriate community services available to cater for the needs of individuals with ID. Different countries have developed various models of care to deal with this shift in responsibility. These models of care include: enhancements, already existing mainstream health care and specialty care programmes, which specifically target the health needs of this population. In England for example, 'community learning disability teams' were created to provide a diverse range of clinical services to meet the comprehensive mental and physical health needs of persons with ID.

There are virtually no documented models or plans in many low and middle-income countries for persons with ID. For example, in Nigeria, the majority of persons with ID are kept in religious and other informal settings away from the opportunity to participate in society. Families often keep children with ID locked up and are ashamed to be identified with them. A major hindrance to the community inclusion of individuals with ID is stigma and discrimination and this also influences access to care and services.

The law and offenders with intellectual disability

Children and adolescents who are under the juvenile justice system (JJS) are found to have higher rates of ID when compared with children in the general population. A study carried out in Ibadan, Nigeria found that almost half (46.7%) of the inmates in the Ibadan Remand Home (custodial part of the JJS in Oyo State, Nigeria) had ID of varying degrees.[39]

Children with ID within the JJS are among the most marginalised. The reasons for this include the changing definitions of ID and offences, the shifting responses of the general population, the reactions of carers, and changes in the JJS and criminal justice system (CJS). All these affect those who are labelled with the term 'intellectually disabled offender'. There is an evidently poor identification of ID offenders by JJS and CJS agencies and inconsistent and inadequate responses by health services, social services and the CJS to the challenge presented by ID offenders.

Legal capacity of individuals with intellectual disability

Decisions in the lives of individuals with ID often generate a significant dilemma in which there is the desire to allow them make their own choices on one hand and the commonly felt need to protect them from making potentially harmful decisions on the other hand. There is often the debate of whether an individual has the capacity to make a decision or not. The Mental Capacity Act (UK) says

> . . . *a person is said to lack capacity in relation to a matter if at the material time he is unable to make a decision for himself in relation to the matter because of an impairment of, or a disturbance in the functioning of the mind or brain.*[40]

The Act also recommends that health professionals have to ask the following questions to establish capacity or the lack of it:

- Can he/she understand the information related to the decision?
- Can he/she remember the information long enough to make a decision?
- Can he/she weigh/analyze the information to reach a decision?
- Can he/she communicate the decision in any way at all, such as talking, using sign language or hand signals, or squeezing someone's hand?

If a person lacks capacity in any of these areas, then this represents a lack of capacity (Mental Capacity Act 2005: Code of Practice).

The Convention on the Rights of Persons with Disabilities (CRPD), adopted by the United Nations General Assembly in December 2006, has significantly affected international human rights law to guaranteeing the equal rights of persons with disabilities. The convention emphasizes the principles of non-discrimination and equality for those with disabilities. There is a gradual shift from the 'medical model' to the 'social model', from assuming that the problems of ID rests with the impairment and the affected individual to viewing the problem of ID as barriers the society erected against people with disabilities.

Article 12 of the CRPD requires that those states that have ratified the treaty recognize that persons with disabilities as having the legal capacity on an equal basis with others in all aspects of life, and that disability alone does not justify the deprivation of legal capacity.

> *Article 12 of the Convention on the Rights of Persons with Disabilities requires State parties to recognize persons with disabilities as individuals before the law, possessing legal capacity, including capacity to act, on an equal basis with others. [...] The centrality of this article in the structure of the Convention and its instrumental value in the achievement of numerous other rights should be highlighted.*

United Nations, General Assembly Human Rights Council (2009), Thematic Study by the Office of the United Nations High Commissioner for Human Rights on enhancing awareness and understanding of the Convention on the Rights of Persons with Disabilities, A/HRC/10/48, 26 January 2009, paragraph 43

It is important to recognize that different degrees of incapacity may exist and that (in)capacity may vary from time to time. Once the legal capacity of a person with ID is totally or partially restricted, a protective measure can be instituted. In most developed countries, this will mean the appointment of a guardian. A guardian will be appointed only if the court bases its judgment on the psychiatric opinion of a qualified and licensed psychiatrist and other evidence. Other terminologies that have been used in different countries to describe a person who is assigned to supervise an individual with ID include trustee, mentor, curator and tutor.

Characteristics of a guardian

   i. He/she should be an adult above 18 years of age
  ii. He/she should be reliable and trustworthy
 iii. He/she should have an appropriate level of skill and competence to carry out the necessary tasks
  iv. He/she should have a close and stable ties with the person
   v. He/she should have legal capacity
  vi. He/she should have no criminal convictions
 vii. He/she should have no conflict of interest in assuming the role.

However, it is imperative to concentrate on enhancing the ability of individuals with ID to make their own decisions. This can be done through:

- Making decision-making a major element in special education curricula
- Implementing habilitation programmes and services for individuals who identify difficulties in making

decisions, and who seek to address and remedy those problems

- Constant provision of necessary information that will help individuals with ID in decision making

Individuals who have ID present unique difficulties in the area of capacity and decision-making. Their interest in autonomous decision making in important areas of their own lives demands greater respect than the law and service delivery system now offer, especially in the developing world.

True autonomy is not promoted by pretending that an individual is competent to make choices that he or she cannot in fact understand. Clinicians and care-givers should also note that competence to make decisions is not an all-or-nothing phenomenon, but rather varies with the complexity and importance of the subject matter that requires decision.

Research gaps in ID in Nigeria and sub-Saharan Africa

Sub-Saharan Africa is home to a large number of persons with ID.[10] There are many challenges facing persons with intellectual disability in this region, among which are the high prevalence of persons with ID, discrimination, and access to justice and education coupled with high poverty levels.[41,10]

Many individuals with ID in sub-Saharan Africa are still being cared for in institutions and majority who attend school are in segregated schools.[8] There is also a high prevalence of preventable causes of intellectual disability in this region.[6]

Few studies have looked into the issue of intellectual disability in Africa[6,10] and majority focussed on cross-sectional community-based epidemiologic studies[42] to determine prevalence rates. There are very few interventional studies in sub-Saharan Africa geared towards improving outcomes for children and adolescents with ID.

A recent interventional study that assessed the impact of training on the social skills of pupils in a 'special school' in southwest Nigeria reported significant improvement in the social skills of the participants. This study showed that it is imperative that information on the epidemiology and burden of disability of ID be recognized; but more importantly, the necessary care and appropriate interventions should be extended to children and adolescents with ID in Africa. More emphasis should be placed on inclusive education systems as enshrined in the Convention on the Rights of Persons with Disabilities[43] of which Nigeria and other countries in sub-Sahara Africa have ratified.

There is a clear need to promote principles of early identification, inclusion, and self-determination of people with ID; efforts should also be made at reducing the occurrence and impact of associated, co-morbid, and secondary conditions. Currently, care givers play very significant roles in the care of individuals in Africa, hence empowering care-givers and family members is a core area of need that requires urgent attention. Promoting healthy behaviour in people with ID and ensuring equitable access to quality health care are important.

Public awareness, education and community-level interventions for reducing the misconceptions and stigma related to ID are needed in addition to culturally sensitive treatment methods to improve attitudes towards and management of ID.[44] Awareness about the causes, early signs and available services should be in the forefront in reducing morbidity and mortality associated with ID.

References

1. World Health Organization (WHO). (1992). Atlas: global resources for persons with intellectual disabilities. Geneva: World Health Organization.

2. American Association of Intellectual and Developmental disability (AAIDD) (2013). Definition of Intellectual Disability. http:/aaidd.org/ intellectual-disability/definition. Accessed 03/12/2013.

3. Harris JC. (2006). Intellectual disability: understanding its development, causes, classification, evaluation, and treatment. Oxford University Press.

4. Carulla LS, Reed GM, Vaez-azizi LM, Cooper SA, Leal R, Bertelli M, Adnams C, Cooray S, Deb S, Dirani LA, Girimaji SC. (2011). Intellectual developmental disorders: towards a new name, definition and framework for "mental retardation/intellectual disability" in ICD-11. *World Psychiatry.* 10(3):175-80.

5. Scior K, Furnham A. (2011). Development and validation of the intellectual disability literacy scale for assessment of knowledge, beliefs and attitudes to intellectual disability. Research in Developmental Disabilities. 32(5):1530-41.

6. Adnams CM. (2010). Perspectives of intellectual disability in South Africa: epidemiology, policy, services for children and adults. *Current Opinion in Psychiatry.* 23:436–440.

7. Durkin M. (2002). The epidemiology of developmental disabilities in low-income countries. *Developmental Disabilities Research Reviews.* 8(3):206-11.

8.   World Health Organization (WHO). (2007). The ICD-10 classification of mental and behavioural disorders: clinical descriptions and diagnostic guidelines. Geneva: World Health Organization.

9.   Mercadante MT, Evans-Lacko S, Paula CS. (2009). Perspectives of intellectual disability in Latin American countries: epidemiology, policy, and services for children and adults. *Current Opinion in Psychiatry*, 22, 469–474.

10. Njenga F (2009). Perspectives of intellectual disability in Africa: epidemiology and policy services for children and adults. *Current Opinion in Psychiatry*, 22(5), p 457-461.

11. Battaglia A. (2011): Sensory impairment in mental retardation: a potential role for NGF. *Archives of Italian Biology*. 149(2): 193-203.

12. Lenroot RH, Gogtay N, Greenstein DK, Wells EM, Wallace GL, Clasen LS, Blumenthal JD, Lerch J, Zijdenbos AP, Evans AC, Thompson PM, Giedd JN.(2007). Sexual dimorphism of brain developmental trajectories during childhood and adolescence. *Neuroimage*, 36: 1065–1073.

13. American Psychiatric Association. Diagnostic and statistical manual of mental disorders (DSM-5). American Psychiatric Pub; 2013 May 22.

14. Kopelowicz A, Liberman RP, Zarate R. (2006). Recent advances in social skills training for schizophrenia. *Schizophrenia Bulletin*, 32(S), S12–S23.

15. Maulik PK, Harbour CK. (2010). Epidemiology of intellectual disability. International *Encyclopedia of Rehabilitation*.

16. Adeniyi Y, Omigbodun O. (2016). Effect of a classroom-based intervention on the social skills of pupils with intellectual disability in Southwest Nigeria. Child and Adolescent Psychiatry and Mental Health.2016, 10:29 DOI: 10.1186/s13034-016-0118-3.

17. Antonacci DJ, Attiah N. (2008): Diagnosis and treatment of mood disorders in adults with Developmental Disabilities. *Psychiatric Quarterly*, 79: 171-192.

18. Matson JL, Shoemaker ME (2011). Psychopathology and intellectual disability. *Current Opinion in Psychiatry*. 24(5):367-71.

19. White P, Chant D, Edwards N, Townsend C, Waghorn G. (2005). Prevalence of intellectual disability and comorbid mental illness in an

Australian community sample. *Australian and New Zealand Journal of Psychiatry.* 39(5):395-400.

20. Baxter H, Lowe K, Houston H, Jones G, Felce D, Kerr M. (2006). Previously unidentified morbidity in patients with intellectual disability. *Br J Gen Pract.* 1;56(523):93-8.

21. Kwok H, Cheung PW. (2007). Co-morbidity of psychiatric disorder and medical illness in people with intellectual disabilities. *Current Opinion in Psychiatry.* 20:443–449.

22. Kerker BD, Owens PL, Zigler E, Horwitz SM. (2004): Mental health disorders among individuals with mental retardation: challenges to accurate prevalence estimates. Public Health Reports. 119: 409–417.

23. Emerson E, Hatton C. (2004). Estimating the current need/demand for supports for people with learning disabilities in England. *Institute for Health Research,* Lancaster University.

24. Sarimski K. (2010). Adaptive skills, behavior problems and parenting stress in mothers of boys with fragile X syndrome. *Journal of Mental Health Research in Intellectual Disabilities.* 3(1).

25. Jansen DE, Krol B, Groothoff JW, Post D. (2006). Towards improving medical care for people with intellectual disability living in the community: possibilities of integrated care. *Journal of Applied Research in Intellectual Disabilities* 19.2: 214-218.

26. Krahn GL, Hammond L, Turner A. (2006). A cascade of disparities: health and health care access for people with intellectual disabilities. *Developmental Disabilities Research Reviews.* 12(1):70-82.

27. May ME, Kennedy CH. (2010). Health and problem behaviour among people with intellectual disabilities. *Behaviour Analysis in Practice.*3(2):4-12.

28. Piazza CC, Fisher WW, Brown KA, Shore BA, Patel MR, Katz RM, Sevin BM, Gulotta CS, Blakely-Smith A. (2003). Functional analysis of inappropriate mealtime behaviours. *Journal of Applied Behaviour Analysis.* 36:187–204.

29. Emerson E, Hatton C. (2007). Mental health of children and adolescents with intellectual disabilities in Britain. *The British Journal of Psychiatry.* 191(6):493-9.

30. Coppus AM, Evenhuis HM, Verberne GJ, Visser FE, Oostra BA, Eikelenboom P, Van Gool WA, Janssens AC, Van Duijn CM. (2008). Survival in elderly persons with Down syndrome. *J Am Geriatr Soc* 56: 2311-2316.

31. Meijer, M. M., S. Carpenter, and F. A. Scholte. (2004). European manifesto on basic standards of health care for people with intellectual disabilities. *Journal of Policy and Practice in Intellectual Disabilities* 1.1 : 10-15.

32. Piachaud, J. (2002). Teaching learning disability to undergraduate medical students. *Advances in Psychiatric Treatment* 8.5: 334-341.

33. Kauffman JM, Hung LY. (2009). Special education for intellectual disability: Current trends and perspectives. *Current Opinion in Psychiatry.* 22(5):452-6.

34. Mansell, J. (2006). The underlying instability in statutory child protection: understanding the system dynamics driving risk-assurance levels. *Social Policy Journal of New Zealand*, 28:97–132.

35. Chataika T. (2012). Disability, development and post-colonialism. In: *Disability and social theory: New developments and directions* Eds Goodley D, Hughes B, Davis L. UK: Palgrave Macmillan, 252-72.

36. Beadle-Brown J, Mansell JL, Whelton B, Hutchinson A, Skidmore C. (2006). People with learning disabilities in 'out-of-area' residential placements: 2. Reasons for and effects of placement. *Journal of Intellectual Disability Research.* 50(11):845-56.

37. Mckenzie JA, Macleod CI. (2012). Rights discourses in relation to education of people with intellectual disability: towards an ethics of care that enables participation. *Disability & Society.* 27(1):15-29.

38. Dessemontet RS, Bless G, Morin D. (2012). Effects of inclusion on the academic achievement and adaptive behaviour of children with intellectual disabilities. *Journal of Intellectual Disability Research.* 56(6):579-87.

39. Atilola O, Omigbodun O, Bella-Awusah T, Lagunju I, Igbeneghu P. (2014). Neurological and intellectual disabilities among adolescents within a custodial institution in South West Nigeria. *Journal of Psychiatric and Mental Health Nursing*, 21(1), 31-38.

40. Mental Capacity Act, 2005. http://www.legislation.gov.uk/ukpga /2005/9/contents

41. Mckenzie JA, McConkey R, Adnams C. (2013). Intellectual disability in Africa: Implications for research and service development. *Disability and Rehabilitation*. 35(20):1750-5.

42. Maulik PK, Darmstadt GL. (2007). Childhood disability in low-and middle-income countries: overview of screening, prevention, services, legislation, and epidemiology. *Pediatrics*.S1-55.

43. United Nations (2006): UN Treaty Collection. Parties to the Convention on the Rights of Persons with Disabilities. (Retrieved 20/12/2013).

44. Balogh R, Ouellette-Kuntz H, Bourne L, Lunsky Y, Colantonio A. (2009).Organising healthcare services for persons with an intellectual disability. *The Cochrane Library*.

Other Selected Readings

Adewumi T. (2015). Child and Adolescent Intellectual Disability. In: *Child Health; Ibadan Medical Specialist Group*. Eds. Lagunju I, Adeyoju AE. Ibadan. BookBuilders Editions Africa. p.359-388.

Ellis JW. (1992). Decisions by and for people with mental retardation: Balancing considerations of autonomy and protection. *Vill. L. Rev.*, 37 (6), 1779.

European Union Agency for Fundamental Rights (2013). Legal Capacity of persons with intellectual disability and persons with mental health problems.

Simeonsson RJ. ICF CY: A universal tool for documentation of disability. *Journal of Policy and Practice in Intellectual Disabilities*. 6.2 (2009): 70-72.

8

Psychoactive Substance Misuse in West Africa

Olawale Lagundoye, Babajide Adeyefa

Introduction

The recreational use of psychoactive substances is fairly common in the society. Alcohol and illicit drug use account for 5.4% of the world's annual disease burden.[1] Addictive disorders are chronic recurring disorders often associated with maladaptive behavioural patterns that have developed over time.

An addiction occurs when an individual's substance use impacts on aspects of that person's well-being, usually with negative consequences in several domains of their existence, including their physical, psychological and social well-being. Addictive disorders are characterized by a cluster of cognitive, behavioural and physiological symptoms, in which the individual continues to use a particular substance(s) despite suffering harmful consequences as a result of their use.

Physiological symptoms include the development of tolerance (the need to consume more of the substance to experience the same effect) and withdrawal symptoms on abstinence, which are relieved by taking more of the substance (for certain substances, some symptoms are less relevant and, in a few instances, such as in the use of inhalants, withdrawal symptoms do not occur).

Behavioural symptoms include craving, inability to stop the use of the substance once its use commences and a relapse to substance misuse after a period of abstinence from the particular substance. In addition to substance-related disorders, there is a growing evidence base for behavioural addictions which present with behavioural symptoms similar to those produced by substance misuse disorders and which have been found to activate reward systems like those activated by drugs of abuse (the evidence being the strongest for a gambling disorder, less so than for other behavioural addictions).

Historical perspective

Psychoactive substance use in sub-Saharan Africa reflects the socioeconomic and political changes in the region through the 20th and early 21st century. Alcoholic beverages had been produced and consumed locally in sub-Saharan Africa for centuries. Ethiopia is one of the world regions where plants useful in alcohol production (barley, millet, maize, etc) were first grown.[2] Alcohol consumption was largely a pastime of middle-aged males, with drinking among women and children restricted.[3,4]

The rapid socioeconomic and cultural transformations across the continent in the 21st century were associated with changes in the patterns of alcohol production and consumption, with drinking becoming more prevalent among the younger age groups.[5] A WHO report[6] in 2001 estimated that Lesotho had the highest increase in per capita consumption of alcohol per adult (15 years and above), with Nigeria being the fifth highest.

Data on the regional prevalence of psychoactive substance use in sub-Saharan Africa is limited by the lack of relevant government policies, poor data collecting systems and limited collation of epidemiological or treatment utilization data. In Nigeria, the substances commonly misused are alcohol, tobacco, cannabis, prescription drugs, non-prescribed hypnotics and cough syrups. In Nigeria, over half of the male respondents had used alcohol and about half of these users had commenced the use by the age of 20.[4] Heavy episodic (binge) drinking and the tendency to drink to intoxication appeared remarkably higher in South Africa, Uganda and Namibia.[3]

Annual cigarette consumption in sub-Saharan Africa remains low relative to other developing countries, but there was a 38.4% increase between 1995 and 2000.[7] The prevalence of tobacco use among women and younger adults has gone up amid concerns that tobacco companies are targeting developing countries to make up for declining markets in developed economies.[8] The most widely produced and consumed illicit drug in Africa is cannabis. Cannabis is not indigenous to West Africa. In places where it grows, it was not a cash crop until the middle to late 20th century, when globalization, war and economic deprivation contributed to these changes.[9,10] It is estimated that 25% of the world's cannabis is grown on the African continent.[11]

The use of cannabis as a recreational drug was initially confined to the soldiers and people of the lower socioeconomic class (migrants, road workers, etc.). It now has a widespread acceptance and use by students in high school and university, as well as professionals in recent years. Between 1962 and 1970, there was a 6.7% increase in the number of cases with cannabis use seen at a neuropsychiatric facility in Lagos, Nigeria.[11] In 2005, the UNODC estimated that about 7.7% of the African population aged 15-64 years were using cannabis, with the highest prevalence in West Africa, Central Africa and Southern Africa. Between 2004 and 2005, 17 African countries reported increasing levels of cannabis use. The cannabis plant is grown in all 36 states of Nigeria, and 70% of the cannabis in South Africa is grown in Lesotho.[11] Cannabis tends to be consumed by smoking, it is also processed into cannabis paste, hashish and added to local alcoholic beverages (*akpeteshie* in Ghana, *jedi* in South-western Nigeria). It is also smoked in a mixture with cocaine or heroin in Nigeria, Ghana, Cameroon and South Africa.[12]

Other drugs abused in sub-Saharan Africa include opiates (heroin, codeine and morphine), amphetamines, cocaine and Khat. Asuni[6] reported that "heroin was practically unknown in Nigeria as a drug of abuse." A UN report in 1983 reiterated that opioid use was not extensive in Africa. In 1987, the United Nations noted the rapid spread of heroin abuse in Mauritius, Nigeria and Somalia, which had gotten worse by the mid-1990s.[13] Recent reports in Nigeria indicate an increase in the misuse of codeine-containing cough syrups, mainly benylin with codeine, tutolin and emzolin (these typically contain 10.95 mg of codeine in a 100ml mixture).

Khat (*Catha edulis*) is indigenous to Eastern Africa, though relatively unknown outside East and North Africa. Its fresh leaves and shoots contain the mild stimulants cathinone and cathine. It was traditionally chewed by elderly men in social gatherings, but more recently used by younger men. It is the third most commonly used psychoactive substance among young people in East Africa and is estimated to be one of Ethiopia's most valuable exports.[3,14] Khat was recently re-categorized as a Class C drug in the UK under the Misuse of Drugs Act 1971 (revised in 2014), to reduce its use and prevent its supply and possession, mainly in displaced immigrants' communities, where its use was becoming problematic.

Aetiology

Factors that predispose individuals to substance misuse include biological factors such as heredity, personality traits, co-morbid mental illness and individual factors such as preference for a particular substance. Societal factors, including unemployment and the local availability of specific substances (the more readily available a substance is, the higher the likelihood of its misuse) are also associated with substance use.

Risk factors for substance misuse peculiar to Africa include political instability, increased availability of drugs (West Africa is a recognized conduit for drug trafficking), high youth unemployment, poor law enforcement, family instability and disruption. Other relevant local factors include poor compliance with regulatory framework for access to prescription drugs and other controlled drugs in many parts of Africa, limited access to psychological interventions for emotional disorders, and limited adoption of and implementation of relevant policies.

Table 1. F10-F9: Mental and behavioural disorders due to psychoactive substance use

ICD10 code	Disorder
F10	Mental and behavioural disorders due to use of alcohol
F11	Mental and behavioural disorders due to use of opioids
F12	Mental and behavioural disorders due to use of cannabinoids
F13	Mental and behavioural disorders due to use of sedatives or hypnotics
F14	Mental and behavioural disorders due to use of cocaine
F15	Mental and behavioural disorders due to use of other stimulants, including caffeine
F16	Mental and behavioural disorders due to use of hallucinogens
F17	Mental and behavioural disorders due to use of tobacco
F18	Mental and behavioural disorders due to use of volatile solvents
F19	Mental and behavioural disorders due to multiple drug use and use of other psychoactive substances

Clinical definitions

The main classification systems — ICD 10 (F10 - 19) and DSM-5 (481) — categorize addictive disorders as disorders due to psychoactive substance use[15] and substance use disorders[16]

Substance use disorders range from mild to severe, and can be classified by descriptive specifiers, such as 'in early remission', 'in sustained remission', 'on maintenance treatment, and 'in a controlled environment'.[15]

An important characteristic of substance use disorders is an underlying change in brain circuits that persists beyond abstinence (detoxification), particularly in individuals with severe disorders. The behavioural effects of these underlying brain changes may be exhibited in the repeated relapses and intense drug craving when the individuals are exposed to drug-related stimuli. These persistent drug effects may benefit from long-term approaches to treatment.

Diagnosis is made following an assessment, comprising a combination of a self-reported history, evidence of clinical signs and symptoms, collaborative information and an objective analysis of the biological specimens of urine, blood, saliva and hair.

Current approaches to treatment

Treatment for addiction involves a number of evidence-based pharmacological and non-pharmacological interventions, adhering to the core principles of:

- Harm reduction
- Engagement
- Specific treatment (to the specific substance of abuse)
- Relapse prevention
- Rehabilitation with individual recovery

Harm reduction interventions include:

- Harm reduction
- Health advice
- Education about specific harms
- Screening and immunization (hepatitis B and C)
- Needle exchange programmes
- Advice about safe sex
- Take home Naloxone
- Pharmacological interventions for opioid dependence, including the misuse of prescription drugs

A critical component of treatment involves behavioural change, and this includes identifying the following three factors:

- Have predisposed the individual to substance use
- Act to maintain continued substance use
- Put the individual at risk of returning to substance use (relapse)

The cycle of change as proposed in the illustration in figure 1 is useful in understanding the stages that an individual passes through during the change process. Each stage is not fixed nor mutually exclusive, and the individual can go through the different stages several times in his/her journey to recovery. The professional should be able to identify where in the cycle of change the individual is utilizing a range of appropriate evidence-based interventions within a therapeutic framework.[16]

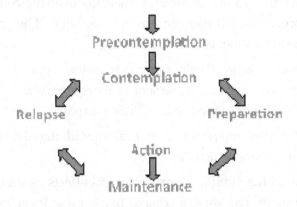

Figure 1. Diagram illustrating the cycle of change.[17]

Pharmacological interventions for psychoactive substance misuse can be broadly put into two categories:

- Substitution or maintenance
- Detoxification or abstinence

Maintenance treatment

In the context of treating opioid dependence, maintenance treatment aims to provide stability by reducing craving, preventing withdrawal, eliminating the hazards of injecting and freeing the individual from preoccupation with obtaining illicit opioids, and enhance overall functioning. The aim is for the individual who is dependent on illicit opioids is to progress from maintenance to detoxification and longer-term abstinence without medication.

Maintenance treatment comprises the prescription of an opiate with a long half-life as a substitute in the treatment of addiction to a range of opiates (heroin, over-the-counter (OTC) preparations, codeine, morphine, etc). The main maintenance treatments for opiates are:

- *Methadone*, a synthetic opioid receptor agonist with pharmacological activity similar to morphine, with a long half-life in comparison to heroin or morphine.

- *Subutex (Buprenorphine)*, a partial opioid agonist with opioid antagonist activity.

- *Suboxone*, has similar pharmacological effects as subutex, but contains naloxone, an opioid blocker that is activated, precipitating an acute opiate withdrawal and triggered if suboxone is injected rather than taken sublingually

Methadone maintenance is most effective when used in conjunction with psychosocial interventions in a structured treatment setting, with the principles of contingency management at its core. In the treatment of opiate addiction, the methadone maintenance treatment is effective, as it helps in reducing substance use and alleviates associated psychiatric illness. The treatment is also associated with reduction in criminal activity (monitored by contact with the criminal justice system), return to employment, improvement in family and social life, and reduction in medical morbidity and the use of other associated services and the cost burden to other systems.

Positive outcomes are found to correlate positively with retention in treatment and the duration of treatment.

Methadone maintenance treatment tends to be long-term (about 5-10 years). It requires a complex system of treatment administration, which includes: supervision, dispensing of methadone, titrations, monitoring of compliance, engagement with psychosocial interventions (aimed at skills acquisition in a bid to achieve competencies for a sustained abstinence from illicit drugs), control to prevent diversion and risk of death to the uninitiated, etc.

Detoxification

Detoxification is the use of a medication to alleviate/minimize the physical symptoms of withdrawal that individuals experience on stopping/discontinuing a substance of abuse. It is related to the rebound phenomenon that occurs at the neuroreceptor levels as a result of withdrawal from a specific substance. The withdrawal phenomena are specific to the individual substances of abuse, though cross tolerance can occur around a number of substances that affect the same group of neuroreceptors.

Detoxification tends to be time limited. It is useful in the treatment of addiction to alcohol, benzodiazepines and opiates, and less effective for substances such as cocaine or cannabis.

• All detoxification programmes require psychosocial interventions as part of the relapse prevention strategies to support a maintained abstinence, post detoxification, in the treatment of addiction to opiates.

- Relapse prevention medications for alcohol dependence include disulfiram, acamprosate, naltrexone, nalmephene and anti-craving blockers.

- The opioid antagonist (naltrexone) can be used to help maintain abstinence post detoxification.

- Not all substances of abuse are associated with withdrawal phenomenon and, as such, not all require detoxification.

For the majority of substances liable to be misused (cocaine, cannabis, Khat and solvents, among others), there are no effective pharmacological interventions available. The main treatment interventions for these consists of a combination of psychosocial and psychological interventions.

Psychosocial interventions

Psychosocial interventions play an important role in the treatment of drug misuse. They aim to support the addicted individual in developing alternative skills useful in maintaining continued abstinence from substance use and also treat associated co-morbidities.

These therapies are important adjuncts to pharmacological treatments and are useful in the treatment of addictions. They include:

- *Brief interventions*: These comprise structured brief advice about the harmful effects of a substance abused purposely for enhancing self-efficacy or self-confidence.

This advice is effective in reducing drug use in non-dependent individuals.

- *Motivational-based approaches*: These include motivational enhancement therapy, and motivational interviewing, aimed at changing an individual's behaviour, improving motivation to change and resolving ambivalence to change.

- *Cognitive behavioural therapy (CBT)*: This aims at changing the drug user's behaviour by changing the way the individual thinks and/or behaves, utilizing cognitive strategies.

- *Relapse prevention*: This treatment approach seeks to identify potential risks and triggers, and develop alternative ways of dealing with them as part of a repertoire of approaches to reduce the risks of returning to substance use. This tends to utilize a CBT approach that encompasses basic learning principles.

- *Contingency management* involves providing the individual with tangible rewards (such as monetary vouchers) to reinforce behavioural change. This is found to be effective in the treatment of cocaine addiction and cannabis use.

Other evidence-based approaches include:

- Behavioural couples therapy
- Network therapy
- Twelve step facilitation programme
- Self-help programmes
- Smart recovery programme

Treatment of co-morbidity

In treating addictive disorders, the management of co-occurring mental disorders and physical illness is important. These include appropriate pharmacological interventions, and a range of psychological interventions which include psychodynamic psychotherapy and mindfulness-based interventions.

Conclusion

Addictive disorders are chronic recurring disorders often associated with maladaptive behavioural patterns that have developed over time. Effective treatment interventions comprise a range of pharmacological and psychosocial interventions relevant to the specific addiction. Behavioural change is common to the treatment approaches, utilizing a number of evidence-based psychological interventions.

Specific factors such as the duration of treatment, the therapeutic alliance, therapist factors such as enhancing positive expectancies, inspiring hope, conveying a deep understanding of the behavioural, cognitive and physiological phenomena that an individual develops after repeated substance use, have been found to be important in an individual's recovery.[18,19]

Learning points and objectives

- The prevalence of substance misuse in sub-Saharan Africa is on the increase. Early identification and harm reduction interventions are important steps in addressing these issues.

- Treatment interventions include pharmacological and non-pharmacological interventions, depending on the substance.

- Behavioural change is essential for treatment to be effective. The 'cycle of change' is a useful framework to assist in formulating the individual's progress and approaches to treatment.

- Relapse prevention is a crucial component of the treatment and should be commenced early in treatment.

References

1. World Health Organization. WHO Report on the Global Tobacco Epidemic: Implementing Smoke-free Environments. World Health Organization, Geneva, 2009.

2. Grant M. *Alcohol and Emerging Markets: Patterns, Problems, and Responses*. Routledge, UK, 2013.

3. Acuda W, Othieno CJ, Obondo A, Crome IB. The epidemiology of addiction in Sub-Saharan Africa: A synthesis of reports, reviews, and original articles. *Am J Addict.* 2011;20(2):87-99.

4. Gureje O, Degenhardt L, Olley B, Uwakwe R, Udofia O, Wakil A, et al. A descriptive epidemiology of substance use and substance use disorders in Nigeria during the early 21st century. *Drug Alcohol Depend.* 2007;91(1):1-9.

5. Kortteinen T. *Agricultural Alcohol and Social Change in the Third World*. Vol. 38. Finnish Foundation for Alcohol Studies, Finland 1989.

6. Jernigan DH, World Health Organization. Global Status Report: Alcohol and Young People. World Health Organization, Geneva, 2001.

7. Oluwafemi A, Shafey O, Dolwick S, Guindon G. *Regional Summary for the African Region. Tobacco Control Country Profiles*. 2nd edition. American Cancer Society, 2003.

8. Townsend L, Flisher AJ, Gilreath T, King G. A systematic literature review of tobacco use among adults 15 years and older in sub-Saharan Africa. *Drug Alcohol Depend.* 2006; 84(1):14-27.

9. Asuni T. The drug abuse scene in Nigeria. *NIDA Res Monogr.* 1978; (19):15-25.

10. Affinnih YH. Revisiting sub-Saharan African countries' drug problems: Health, social, economic costs, and drug control policy. *Subst Use Misuse* 2002; 37(3):265-90.

11. UNODC. Cannabis in Africa. United Nations Office on Drugs and Crime, Vienna, 2007.

12. ODCCP. Nexus in Africa. United Nations, Vienna, 1999.

13. International Narcotics Control Board. Availability of Opiates for Medical Needs. United Nations, New York, 1995.

14. Manghi RA, Broers B, Khan R, Benguettat D, Khazaal Y, Zullino DF. Khat use:Llifestyle or addiction? *J Psychoactive Drugs* 2009; 41(1):1-10.

15. WHO. *The ICD-10 Classification of Mental and Behavioural Disorders: Clinical Descriptions and Diagnostic Guidelines*. World Health Organization, Geneva. 1992.

16. American Psychiatric Association. *Diagnostic and Statistical Manual of Mental Disorders*. 5th edition. American Psychiatric Association, Washington, 2013.

17. Prochaska JO, DiClemente CC.. Transtheoretical therapy: Toward a more integrative model of change. *Psychotherapy: Theory Research & Practice* 1982; 19(3): 276-288.

18. Project MATCH Research Group. Matching alcohol treatments to Client heterogenicity: post treatment drinking outcomes. *Journal of Studies on Alcoholism* 1997; 58: 7-29.

19. UK Alcohol Treatment Trial. Effectiveness of treatment for alcohol problems findings of the randomised UK alcohol treatment trail (UKATT). *BMJ* 2005; 331: 541-547

Selected readings

Acuda SW, Sebit MB. Prevalence of psychoactive substance use among psychiatric in-patients in Harare, Zimbabwe. *Cent Afr J Med.* 1997;43(8): 226-9.

NICE. Drug misuse in over 16s: Ppsychosocial Interventions. NICE Clinical Guidelines 51. National Collaborating Centre for Mental Health, UK, 2007.

Kanyoni M, Gishoma D, Ndahindwa V. Prevalence of psychoactive substance use among youth in Rwanda. *BMC Res Notes* 2015; 8: 190.

Klein A. Have a piss, drink ogogoro, smoke igbo, but don't take gbana-- hard and soft drugs in Nigeria: A critical comparison of official policies and the view on the street. *J Psychoactive Drugs* 2001; 33(2):111-9.

NICE. Methadone and Buprenorphine for the Management of Opioid Dependence. Technological Appraisal Guidance. National Collaborating Centre for Mental Health, UK, 2007.

Ohaeri JU, Odejide OA. Admissions for drug and alcohol-related problems in Nigerian psychiatric care facilities in one year. *Drug and Alcohol Dependence* 1993; 31(2):101-9.

Onifade PO, Somoye EB, Ogunwobi OO, Ogunwale A, Akinhanmi AO, Adamson TA. A descriptive survey of types, spread and characteristics of substance abuse treatment centers in Nigeria. *Subst Abuse Treat Prev Policy* 2011; 6:25.

Chatter R, Cooper K, Day E, Knight M, Lagundoye O, Wong R, Kaltenthaler E. Psychological and psychosocial interventions for cannabis cessation in adults: a systematic review. *Addiction Research & Theory* 2016; 24(2): 93-110.

Simpson DD, Joe GW, Brown BS. Treatment retention and follow up outcomes in the drug abuse treatment outcomes study. *Pschol Addict Behav* 1997; 11:294-307.

Weich L, Pienaar W. Occurrence of comorbid substance use disorders among acute psychiatric inpatients at Stikland Hospital in the Western Cape, South Africa. *Afr J Psychiatry (Johannesbg)* 2009; 12(3):213-7.

WHO. Global Status report on Alcohol and Health. World Health Organization, Geneva, 2014.

9

Management of Older Adult Mental Health Conditions in sub-Saharan Africa

Olugbenga Akande, Abel A. Ojagbemi, Olusegun Baiyewu

Background

The number of older persons living in sub-Saharan Africa (SSA) is projected to increase by 239% between 2015 and 2050.[1] The rising demographics present several challenges for both mental and physical health services provision in the region. For example, while there is an increase in the burden of conditions such as dementia in SSA[1], specific and implementable policies for the health and well-being of older adults are rare in most countries in the region. There were no geriatric assessment units in Nigeria in the year 2002[2] and little has changed since then, with only one such unit in the University College Hospital, Ibadan. The same is true of most sub-Saharan Africa except, probably, South Africa.[3]

Inadequacies in mental health provision in Africa can be viewed from two angles: poverty and lack of policy. Per capita health expenditure is low in many SSA countries; in the year 2014 it was 17 US dollars in Central Africa Republic, Kenya $78, Ghana $58, Nigeria $118 and South Africa $570. The overall amount for sub-Sahara Africa was $98.[4] These figures are inexplicably low compared with Canada $5292, Switzerland $9674. The World Alzheimer's Report[5] clearly pointed out the relationship between mental health provision for older adults and per capita health expenditure. It thus follows that to some extent there is a relationship between good economic status and provision of good health services.

Also, only a minority of pensionable persons are able to access their pension. There are no social welfare packages, and access to health care is mostly dictated by personal financial resources.[6]

In this chapter we will provide an overview of the current trends in the management of mental health disorders in the older population, and within the unique social, economic and cultural context of SSA.

1. Challenges in managing older people's mental health

Mental health disorders in older adults could present unique challenges in diagnoses and management. As such, clinical practice of old age psychiatry requires skills that bridge the gaps between psychiatry, general medicine/geriatrics, neurology and psychopharmacology.

Differences in clinical presentation between the older and younger person may include the presence of mental and physical health co-morbidities. This overlap may conflate signs and symptoms of one condition with that of another and lead to a more complicated clinical picture. It is thus often important to get collateral information from carers and other close relatives, neighbours or friends.

Co-occurrence of physical and mental health conditions also serves to complicate the management of mental health condition in the older person. First, elderly persons with co-morbidities are also more likely to have greater disability which in turn compounds the management of the mental health disorder. Second, the older person with co-morbidities is also likely to use multiple medications or receive other therapies. Whereas, age-related reductions in hepatic metabolism and reductions in renal drug clearance make older people more likely to be susceptible to the effects of these medication.[7]

In the particular context of SSA, mental health disorders are still poorly understood. Many of the important signs and symptoms of emerging neurobehavioural and emotional disorders are often interpreted in terms of the prevailing socio-cultural beliefs. For example, symptoms such as worsening memory, slowing of function and a lack of spontaneity are perceived as normal and inevitable aspects of aging; whereas hallucinations and delusions are sometimes interpreted as demonic,[8] and many patients with these presentations are ultimately accused of witchcraft or demon possession. These explanatory models, coupled with the prevailing intergenerational living arrangements in many African societies, prevent large numbers of patients from presenting for diagnosis and treatment in the earlier stages of disease.

In most situations of emerging mental health conditions, family members simply take over the everyday responsibilities of their wards, and only present them at the hospital when their behaviour becomes too bewildering to cope with at home.

2. Assessment and treatment of cognitive disorders

Dementia is one of the major causes of disability in older people. It is a complex syndrome characterized by an acquired global, mostly irreversible, and progressive decline of intellect, memory, personality, and ability to cope with activities of daily life, occurring without impairment of consciousness. Dementia runs a chronic course, and is associated with severe adverse consequences on social participation, physical activities and quality of life.

In cognitive impairment (no dementia) and mild cognitive impairment, the cognitive deficit is often less severe than in dementia and normal daily function and independence are generally maintained. Mild cognitive impairment may sometimes precede dementia, and this is observed to be so in up to one third of cases.[9,10]

The most common type of dementia is Alzheimer's disease, followed by vascular dementia (caused by cerebro-vascular/stroke disease); dementia with Lewy body (associated with Parkinson's disease); Parkinson's disease dementia (a separate condition from Lewy body dementia); fronto-temporal dementia (Pick's disease). In sub-Saharan Africa, HIV-related dementia, which is a disease of younger adults not just older people, is of clinical importance.

The flagship of dementia research is the Indianapolis-Ibadan research study[11,12] which reported low prevalence and incidence of dementia in Nigeria. Similar findings have been reported in other studies in Nigeria.[13,14] Some studies from Central African Republic and Tanzania have reported higher prevalence rates.[15,16] The prevalence of dementia generally rises exponentially with age up to the age of 85 years.[11,12] Many studies in the Western world suggest that regular physical exercise and a healthy diet, control of cardiovascular risk factors, such as high blood pressure, lipid levels, blood sugar, weight, alcohol intake and smoking, can reduce the chances of developing dementia. In a recent report, the incidence of dementia decreased in Indianapolis while it remained stable in Ibadan over about 10 years.[17]

A possible explanation for that is the increased awareness in American society which has allowed both individuals and health-care facilities to take appropriate preventive strategies as indicated above. Prince in a global survey suggested that there is some evidence that the incidence of dementia is decreasing in the industrialized world, while the prevalence rate is increasing in East Asia and that is consistent with a worsening cardiovascular risk factor profile.[18]

The most commonly cited risk factors for dementia in the context of SSA include older age and female gender,[12,13,14] hypertension,[19] poor pre-dementia cognitive function and unskilled lifetime occupational attainment.[20]

HIV-associated dementia

Neurocognitive disorders in people with HIV may be caused by the virus directly damaging the brain. They may also be the result of a weakened immune system enabling infections to damage the brain. Countries in sub-Saharan Africa are among the highest contributors to the global HIV burden.

HIV-associated dementia affects younger adults but there may be an increase in older HIV/AIDS survivors on highly active anti-retroviral drugs. Older adults may particularly be at risk of HIV-associated dementia. Reports from SSA gave the prevalence of HIV-associated dementia at between 7% and 38% among HIV clinic attendees.[21,13]

Clinical features and management of dementia syndromes

There are clinical features common to all the dementia syndromes, irrespective of the primary cause of the disease. These include memory loss, which usually presents gradually over time, but can occasionally be abrupt (for instance as a consequence of an acute stroke) with disturbances in new learning and learning capacity, aphasia (language difficulties), apraxia (difficulties with motor movements), agnosia (inability to recognise people/objects), loss of executive function, difficulties in thinking, orientation, comprehension and judgement.

Consciousness is usually not clouded unlike in delirium. In addition, patients with dementia can present with neuropsychiatric features called behavioural and psychological symptoms of dementia (BPSD), including psychotic symptoms such as delusions and hallucinations, repetitive behaviour, mood disturbance (e.g. depression), agitation, wandering, physical aggression, sleep disturbance and disinhibition.[22]

In the studies conducted in Ibadan, Nigeria, depression was the most common behavioural symptom in the context of dementia and mild cognitive impairment.[23] The two most important stages for the clinician to follow in the diagnostic process are:

    i.   To establish a diagnosis of dementia, and

   ii.   To establish the cause of the dementia syndrome.

This will help to both guide management strategies and rule out treatable confounding illnesses such as depression and delirium.

Investigations

Table 1. Assessments to be made in dementia

Clinical history: cognitive, behavioural and psychological symptoms (family history as well as input from close informants/carers)
Physical examination: causes of cognitive impairment (eg. urinary tract infection, cardiac failure, visual or hearing impairment)
Executive functioning: check for impairment of
Activities of daily living : (including washing, dressing, eating)
Medication review
Full blood count (FBC),erythrocyte sedimentation rate (ESR), liver **Function test** (TFT), thyroid function test. Fasting blood sugar, vitamin B_{12} and folate, calcium, fasting lipids
Scans: Computed tomography scan or magnetic resonance imaging

If indicated
Chest X-ray, electrocardiogram (ECG), mid-steam urine (MCS), serology for HIV, syphilis electroencephalogram

Special Investigation
Neuropsychological assessment: These include Consortium to Establish a Registry for Alzheimer's Disease (CERAD)[24]   **Cambridge Cognition Examination (CAMCOG)**[25]   **Clock Drawing Test**[26]   **Mini Mental State Examination MMSE**[27]   In the context of low literacy as observed in the sub-Saharan region, **Stick Design Test**[28] might be useful.

Treatment for dementia

Treatment for dementia can be divided according to the stage of dementia (early stage, middle stage or late stage), sub-divided into pharmacological and non-pharmacological treatment, and further sub-divided into treatments for cognitive symptoms and treatments for non-cognitive symptoms.

People with mild to moderate Alzheimer's disease, dementia with Lewy bodies, and mixed dementia (caused by both Alzheimer's disease and vascular dementia) could benefit from taking a cholinesterase inhibitor. Cholinesterase inhibitors are not a cure, but can treat some symptoms in some patients. They are not licensed for treating any other form of dementia.

There are three cholinesterase inhibitors licensed to treat Alzheimer's: Donepezil (Aricept), Rivastigmine (Exelon) and Galantamine (Reminyl). All three drugs work in a similar way. So far, no difference in the effectiveness of the three cholinesterase inhibitors has been shown, but some people may seem to respond better to one drug than another or have fewer side effects. Rivastigmine is also available in liquid form or in patches, where the drug is absorbed through the skin. People with mild or moderate Alzheimer's disease may find that their conditions improve by taking a cholinesterase inhibitor. This could be improvement in thinking, memory, communication or day-to-day activities. Others may find that their condition stays the same.

Cholinesterase inhibitors work by blocking the enzyme responsible for the breakdown of acetylcholine in the brain. Acetylcholine is the main neurotransmitter for memory, but this treatment option will not stop the disease from progressing in the brain and symptoms can continue to get worse over time. However, they can help people to function at a slightly higher level than they would do without the drug. The most common side effects of cholinesterase inhibitors are nausea (sickness), vomiting, diarrhoea, insomnia, muscle cramps, and tiredness. These effects are often mild and usually only temporary.

Memantine is a partial *N-methyl-D-aspartate* (NMDA) receptor antagonist currently recommended for people with severe Alzheimer's disease, and for people with moderate Alzheimer's if cholinesterase inhibitors don't help or are not suitable. Memantine prevents the excitotoxic actions of glutamate by blocking the influx of calcium ions into the neuron, slowing down cell damage. It is normally given as tablets, but it is also available as a liquid.

Managing behavioural and psychological symptoms of dementia

Behavioural and psychological symptoms of dementia (BPSD) affects between 70% and 90% of individuals with dementia and is of significant distress to both the individual and their care givers.[23,29]

Non-pharmacological management is considered first line in the management of dementia with or without BPSD and should be employed regardless of whether a decision is taken to commence medication. Routine monitoring and evaluation need to be undertaken on a regular basis by the clinician. These strategies are listed.

Non-pharmacological management strategies

- Provide a 'dementia-safe' and friendly environment
- Maintain a set routine
- Avoid over-stimulation
- Psychoeducation for family/care-givers
- Adequate training for care-givers
- Reminders and repetition of information
- Orientation with clocks, calendars, newspapers
- Regular social interaction and activity
- Regular exercise
- Reminiscence therapy
- Validation therapy
- Resolution therapy
- Pet therapy
- Respite care to relieve care-giver burden
- Supportive counselling for family members

A recent study from Tanzania indicates that cognitive stimulation therapy produces substantial improvements in cognition, anxiety, and behaviour symptoms with smaller improvements in quality of life measures in persons with dementia.[30]

A number of individuals with dementia may require pharmacotherapy for the treatment of BPSD. Antipsychotics have traditionally been the treatment of choice for the management of behavioural disturbance in dementia but recent warnings of the increased risk of stroke in elderly patients using all classes of antipsychotics and risk of worsening confusion in dementia now make these drugs second line treatments. A useful approach when deciding on an appropriate agent would be to first identify and treat depression and anxiety disorders if present, secondly to consider cognitive enhancers where appropriate, and finally to consider alternative agents, e.g., anticonvulsants, and antipsychotics (see table 2).

Table 2. Pharmacological therapies in elderly patients

Therapy	Medication	Additional notes
Antidepressants	Citalopram 20mg/day: initiate at 10mg	Few CYP450 interactions
	Fluoxetine 20 - 40mg/day	Inhibits CYP450 2D6 & 3A4 Some dopaminergic activity
SSRIs	Sertraline 50- 100mg	
SARI (serotonin 2 antagonist/ reuptake	Amitriptyline initial dose 25 - 50mg/day, increase gradually to	Cardiotoxic, anticholinergic, antihistaminic side-effects

inhibitor) TCAs	100mg/day Trazodone 25mg at night	Hypotension Antihistaminic side-effects Hypotension
Cholinesterase inhibitors	Donepezil 5 - 10mg at night Galantamine 16-24mg/day Rivastigmine 6 - 12mg in 2 doses	GIT side-effects are common in all three
NMDA receptor antagonist	Memantine 10 mg twice daily	Dizziness and headache may occur
Anticonvulsants	Sodium valproate 10 - 15mg/kg in divided doses Carbamazepine 400mg/day in divided doses	Start with smaller dose and titrate up CYP450 3A4 inducer
Anti-psychotics Typical Atypical	Haloperidol 0.5 - 1mg/day Risperidone 0.5mg twice daily: may initiate at 0.25mg twice daily Quetiapine 25 - 50mg at night Olanzapine 2.5-10mg/day	Watch for EPSEs Weight gain, may increase prolactin Hypotension, sedation, weight gain Weight gain

Management of depression in older people

Depression is a common disorder in older adults. The prevalence of depression in elderly people has been reported to be between 10 and 20%. Older adults with physical illnesses or living in residential care facilities showed a higher prevalence rate of depression. Generally, physical illnesses are associated with an increased risk of depression and depression is significantly more common in people with chronic illnesses than in people who are in good physical health.[31] Depression is generally associated with an increased risk of suicide, decline in functioning and quality of life. It also increases the utilisation of health-care services.

The prevalence rates of depression in older adults in sub-Saharan Africa vary depending on location and method-ology. Studies where depressive symptoms are measured tend to report higher rates than those in which a categorical diagnosis based on ICD-10 or DSM-IV are used. Some of the studies in Nigeria include that of Uwakwe[32] in older adult in-patients; Gureje[33] a community-based study in urban and rural areas; and Sokoya and Baiyewu[34] in older adults attending primary care. Others include those of Baiyewu,[35] of older adults living in rural areas and Olagunju[36] which looks at the burden of depression and social support. A report from South Africa by Tomita[37] examined depression and disability in older adults.

Depression is generally associated with an increased risk of suicide, decline in functioning and quality of life. It also increases the utilisation of health-care services. There are no reports of suicide rates in the older adults in sub-Saharan Africa but suicidal ideas, plans and attempts were 4.0%, 0.7% and 0.2% respectively in community dwellers 65 years or older.[38]

Compared with non-depressed people, those with a 12-month diagnosis had a worse overall quality of life. There is also a high level of unmet needs for treatment of depression in older people. One Nigerian survey found only about 37% of elderly persons with lifetime depression had ever received any form of treatment, either from orthodox or traditional health providers for their depressive illness, with men more likely to have ever done so. Area of residence was related to access to treatment, with those in urban areas three times as likely to have received treatment as those in rural areas.[33]

Many developed countries recommend screening for depression in primary care settings. This is because detection of depression in older adults is difficult, as somatic symptoms of depression such as loss of appetite, weight loss, decreased energy and disturbed sleep are similar to the symptoms of other physical illnesses. However, devoting time to screening in a busy clinic in sub-Saharan Africa may be difficult. Despite all of these complex interactions, depressive illnesses are fairly easy to treat and the cost of treatment is relatively low.

A wide range of pharmaceutical treatments and psychosocial interventions can relieve the symptoms of depression especially if detected and treated early. Early detection and management of the disease can alter the prognosis.

Management options

Screening

Screening for depressive symptoms by use of questionnaires should not be routine, but may be needed in certain clinical situations. Questionnaires that have been proved useful in research situations are ideal. They include the Geriatric Depression Scale (GDS-15 items).[39] There are shorter versions GDS-6 and GDS-5. Another questionnaire that is useful for adults and older adults is Patient Health Questionnaire (PHQ-9). It is a 9 item questionnaire.[40] A shorter form, PHQ-2, is available and can be administered before either PHQ-9 or GDS.15. These questionnaires can easily be filled out by patients, but with the situation of low literacy in the SSA, it might be necessary to have the interviewer administer.

Psychological and talking therapies

There is good evidence for the effectiveness of a number of psycho-social interventions such as cognitive behavioural therapy (CBT), behavioural activation and problem solving treatment. These should be tried before or along with the use of medication (as appropriate) depending on the severity of the depression.

Medication

Antidepressant drugs are equally effective. The principles of prescribing antidepressants are the same as those for prescribing for younger people. First line treatment should be with an SSRI (selective serotonin reuptake inhibitor). Choice of antidepressant should be guided by the patient's previous experience of an antidepressant, and by co-morbidities and side effects.

Tricyclic antidepressants (TCAs) and Serotonin and Noradrenaline reuptake inhibitors (SNRIs) should not be initiated in primary care, but are occasionally suggested for secondary care for use in treatment-resistant depression. Amitriptyline is frequently started in primary care for older people with chronic pain, but co-prescribing of both a TCA and an SNRI should be avoided. At least four weeks of one antidepressant should be tried (and concordance ensured) before changing to another SSRI or an antidepressant of a different class.

The side effects with SSRIs include insomnia, agitation, headache, sexual dysfunction, gastrointestinal disorders (including GI bleeding) so care must be taken if the patient is prescribed aspirin). Antidepressants should be continued for at least six months. Long term treatment for relapse prevention should be considered in people who have had recurrent depression. The use of mood stabilisers and electroconvulsive therapy for severe treatment resistant depression follows the same principles in treating younger adults.

Recognising and treating delirium/acute confusional states

Delirium is characterised by abrupt onset and fluctuating disturbances of cognition (memory, orientation, language skills, mood, thinking), perception, motor behaviour, and the sleep wake cycle.

Delirium is encountered in all health-care settings but probably more so, in non-psychiatric settings. In a study in the United Kingdom, delirium in hospital patients was associated with infections, falls and incontinence. It affected a fifth of acute medical admissions and a third of those aged ≥75 years, and was associated with increased mortality, institutionalisation and dependency over a two year follow-up period.[41]

In Africa, a recent Nigerian study found rates of delirium as high as 18%. Delirium was found in 21.4% of referrals from general medical outpatients, 17.7% of referrals from private hospitals, and 31.6% from the accident and emergency department.[42] Delirium, however, seems to carry an especially grave prognosis in Africa. However in a recent follow up study among post stroke patients in Ibadan, 33 of 99 patients with a mean age of 61 years had delirium. Of those with delirium 65.6% had the hypoactive type, 21.9% hyperactive and 12.1% mixed. At a three- month follow up, 24 had died and 11 others were lost to follow up. Severity of stroke was associated with delirium mortality and dementia.[43]

Despite its public health importance, delirium can be under diagnosed or misdiagnosed, cases often being construed as non-organic mental illnesses or being given no diagnosis. The core cognitive disturbance is impaired attention. The symptoms of delirium may result in agitation at night and drowsiness during the day. However, the presentation varies, ranging from the floridly agitated, hyper-alert, hyperactive patient to the drowsy, hypo-alert patient sleeping quietly in their bed.

Many patients have a mixture of symptoms including inattention, varying degrees of consciousness, hallucinations and delusions. Hypo-alertness in patients is often mistaken for dementia, resulting in delayed or missed opportunities for therapeutic intervention.

It is thought that multiple aetiologies and mechanisms may converge to alter brain function and produce the characteristic symptoms of delirium. Risk factors for delirium include dementia, older age, multiple co-morbidities, psychoactive medication use, sleep deprivation, dehydration, immobility, pain, sensory impairment and hospitalisation.

Delirium is closely linked to dementia—each is a risk factor for the other—and it is now recognised that delirium can cause irreversible decline in cognitive and physical function, as well as increased mortality and nursing home placement.

Most individuals had delirium due to infections, with gastrointestinal infections being the most common source with reports that 73.1% of those with typhoid fever had delirium. It is therefore imperative that psychiatrists in sub-Saharan Africa are vigilant for infectious diseases in patients presenting with confusion, as well as the importance of training health professionals in these environments to recognise and treat delirium.[42]

M	metabolic – hyponatraemia, hypoglycaemia, hypoxaemia
I	infective – urinary tract infection, pneumonia
S	structural – subarachnoid haemorrhage, urinary retention
T	toxic – drugs (e.g. digoxin, lithium) or poisons
E	environmental – being in hospital or the emergency department

Box 1. MISTE: a mnemonic for possible causes of delirium.[44]

Management

Screening and diagnosis

The crucial, and unfortunately, often missing step in delirium management is diagnosis. Given the large and increasing number of older patients in hospital, screening for delirium should become part of routine observations, at least for high-risk patients. However, some training of staff is required. It is very useful, when unsure if a patient's poor cognitive status is new or pre-existing, to ask their family or carer whether they are usually like this.

Further management

Once delirium is identified, initial management aims to detect and treat underlying medical and surgical causes. The list of possible causes is long, and the simple mnemonic MISTE serves as an aide-memoire to categorize potential causes (see box 1 above). A comprehensive assessment including history, examination and appropriate investigations is required when delirium is detected, because many older patients have more than one diagnosis contributing to their delirium.

Appropriate management of the underlying condition(s) and the drugs that the patient is taking, remains the mainstay of delirium treatment. A thorough medication review is important. Anticholinergics, psychoactive medications (including antiepileptic and pain medications), and NSAIDs may also contribute to delirium. Even drugs that are used to treat delirium, particularly if given in excess, can prolong or worsen delirium. It is also important to enquire about over-the-counter and complementary medications, which have marked anticholinergic properties, as these may precipitate delirium.

Hospital Elder Life Program

The Hospital Elder Life Program (HELP) addresses six of the risk factors for delirium, namely cognitive impairment, sleep deprivation, immobility, dehydration and visual and hearing impairment. The program recommends the following:[44]

- reorient and mobilise the patient
- reduce sensory deprivation

- ensure the patient is hydrated
- implement a non-pharmacologic sleep regimen
- limit catheters and restraints

Patients with hyperactive delirium

Managing a patient with hyperactive delirium can be a challenge on any ward. Restraints should be avoided, as they aggravate delirium, as well as increase injuries and falls. Where suitable, asking family to be present as much as possible, even organising a roster of relatives, generally helps to calm agitated patients.

It is important to prevent complications so, for example, agitated patients who keep climbing out of bed may be nursed on low beds or mattresses placed on the floor. It is preferable to allow an agitated patient to pace around a secure delirium ward than to sedate them as this can lead to hypostatic pneumonia or pressure sores.

Use of medication in the management of delirium

Drug therapy is reserved for patients who are at risk of harming themselves or others, for example by pulling out essential medical devices or lines.

Antipsychotics

If drugs are needed, antipsychotics are generally accepted as first-line, except in delirium tremens (caused by alcohol withdrawal). Suggested initial doses are haloperidol 2.5mg, risperidone 0.5mg or olanzapine 2.5mg. Depending on the response, additional doses can be given after 2–4 hours, otherwise daily. However, for more frequent dosing, the patient should be closely monitored for over-sedation.

Treatment of psychotic and other disorders

There are three causes of psychotic illnesses in older people. These are:

- Disorders that have started in adult life and persist into old age, such as schizophrenia, mania and depressive psychosis.
- Psychotic disorders starting after the age of 65 years (such as late onset schizophrenia or paraphrenia)
- Organic psychoses (seen in dementia or delirium)

Treatments for these as well as other common conditions including anxiety and somato form disorders follow the same principles described for younger adults, remembering the essential aphorism of geriatric pharmacology: start low and go slow.

Conclusions

It is important to pay attention to the mental health of older adults in sub-Saharan Africa in clinical service, research and teaching of health practitioners of all categories. This is because of the need for a multidisciplinary approach that is required in the management in geriatrics and psycho-geriatrics. In sub-Saharan Africa in particular there is a dearth of infrastructure and personnel in the subspecialty . This chapter hope to fill some of the learning gaps for those practising in the sub-specialty.

References

1. World Alzheimer Report (2015). The global impact of dementia: an analysis of prevalence, incidence cost and trend. Alzheimer Disease International-2015.

2. Akanji BO, Ogunniyi A, Baiyewu O.(2002). Health care for the older person, a country profile: Nigeria. *Journal of American Geriatric Society* 50:1289-1292.

3. Kalula SZ, Ferreira M, Thomas KG, de Villiers L, Joska JA, Geffen LN. (2010). Profile and management of patients at a memory clinic. *S Afr Med J*; 100(7):449-51.

4. World Development Indicators: Health System: World Bank-http//data.worldbank.org/indicator/SH/XPD/PCAP-Accessed 24/7/2017.

5. World Alzheimer Report (2016). Improving healthcare for people living with dementia: coverage, quality and costs now and in the future-2016.

6. Uwakwe R, Ibeh CC, Modebe AI, Bo E, Ezeama N, Njelita I, Ferri CP, Prince MJ .(2009). The epidemiology of dependence in older people in Nigeria prevalence determinants, informal care, and health service utilization. A 10/66 dementia research group cross-sectional survey. *J Am Geriatr Soc*, 57(9): p. 1620-7.

7. Gureje O, Kola, Ademola A, Olley BO. (2009). Profile, comorbidity and impact of insomnia in the Ibadan study of ageing. *Int J Geriatr Psychiatry*, 24(7): p. 686-93.

8. Uwakwe R.(2000a). Knowledge of religious organizations about dementia and their role in care. *Int J Geriatr Psychiatry*, 15(12): 1152-3.

9. Baiyewu O, Unverzagt FW, Ogunniyi A, Hall KS, Gureje O, Gao S, Lane KA, Hendrie HC.(2002). Cognitive impairment in community-dwelling older Nigerians: clinical correlates and stability of diagnosis. *Eur J Neurol.*; 9(6):573-80.

10. Paddick SM, Kisoli A, Samuel M, Higginson J, Gray WK, Dotchin CL, Longdon AR, Teodorczuk A, Chaote P, Walker RW.(2015a). Mild cognitive impairment in rural Tanzania: prevalence, profile, and outcomes at 4-year follow-up. *Am J Geriatr Psychiatry.*; 23(9):950-9. doi: 10.1016/j.jagp.2014.12.005. Epub 2014 Dec 11.

11. Hendrie HC, Osuntokun BO, Hall KS, Ogunniyi AO, Hui SL, Unverzagt FW, Gureje O, Rodenberg CA, Baiyewu OA, Musick BS, Adeyinka A, Farlow MR, Oluwole SO, Class CA, Komolafe O, Brashear A, Burdine V. (1996). Prevalence of Alzheimer's disease and dementia in two communities: Nigerian Africans and African Americans. *American Journal of Psychiatry*, 152,1485- 1492.

12. Hendrie HC, Ogunniyi A, Hall KS, Baiyewu O, Unverzagt FW, Gureje O, Gao S, Evans RM, Ogunseyinde AO, Adeyinka AO, Musick B, Hui SL.(2001). Incidence of dementia and Alzheimer disease in 2

communities: Yoruba residing in Ibadan, Nigeria, and African Americans residing in Indianapolis, Indiana. *JAMA*. ;285(6):739

13. Yusuf AJ, Baiyewu O, Sheikh TL, Shehu AU.(2011). Prevalence of dementia and dementia subtypes among community-dwelling elderly people in northern Nigeria. *Int Psychogeriatr*.;23(3):379-86.doi:10.1017/S1041610210001158. Epub 2010 Aug 18.

14. Gureje O, Ogunniyi A, Kola L, Abiona T. (2011). Incidence of and risk factors for dementia in the Ibadan study of aging. *J Am Geriatr Soc*, 59(5): 869-74.

15. Guerchet MI, M'belesso P, Mouanga AM, Bandzouzi B, Tabo A, Houinato DS, Paraïso MN, Cowppli-Bony P, Nubukpo P, Aboyans V, Clément JP, Dartigues JF, Preux PM. (2010). Prevalence of dementia in elderly living in two cities of Central Africa: the EDAC survey. *Dement Geriatr Cogn Disord*.; 30(3):261-8. doi: 10.1159/000320247. Epub 2010 Sep 16.

16. Longdon AR, Paddick SM, Kisoli A, Dotchin C, Gray WK, Dewhurst F, Chaote P, Teodorczuk A, Dewhurst M, Jusabani AM, Walker R. (2013). The prevalence of dementia in rural Tanzania: a cross-sectional community-based study. *Int J Geriatr Psychiatry*.

17. Gao S, Ogunniyi A, Hall KS, Baiyewu O, Unverzagt FW, Lane KA, Murrell JR, Gureje O, Hake AM, Hendrie HC.(2016). Dementia incidence declined in African-Americans but not in Yoruba. *Alzheimers Dement*.; 12(3):244-51. doi:10.1016/j.jalz.2015.06.1894. Epub 2015 Jul 26.

18. Prince M, Ali GC, Guerchet M, Prina AM, Albanese E and Wu Y. (2016). Recent global trends in the prevalence and incidence of dementia, and survival with dementia. *Alzheimer's Research & Therapy* 8:23.

19. Ogunniyi A, Lane KA, Baiyewu O, Goa S, Gureje O, Unverzagt FW, Murrel JK, Smith-Gamble V, Hall KS, Hendrie HC. (2011). Hypertension

and incident dementia in community dwelling elderly Yoruba, Nigerians. *Acta Neurologica Scandinavica* 124:396-402.

20. Ojagbemi A, Bello T, Gureje O. (2016). Cognitive reserve, incident dementia and associated mortality in the Ibadan study of ageing. *J Am Geriatr Soc*, 64(3): 590-5.

21. Lawler K, Mosepele M, Ratcliffe S, Seloilwe E, Steele K, Nthobatsang R, Steenhoff A. (2010). Neurocognitive impairment among HIV-positive individuals in Botswana: a pilot study. *J Int AIDS Soc*. 20;13:15. doi: 10.1186/1758-2652-13-15.

22. Cummings JL, Mega M, Gray K, Rosenberg-Thompson S, Carusi DA, Gorrnbein J. (1994). The neuropsychiatric inventory: comprehensive assessment of psychopathology in dementia. *Neurology, 44*, 2308-2314.

23. Baiyewu O, Unverzagt FW, Ogunniyi A, Smith-Gamble V, Gureje O, Lane KA, Gao S, Hall KS, Hendrie HC. (2012). Behavioural symptoms in community-dwelling elderly Nigerians with dementia, mild cognitive impairment, and normal cognition. *Int J Geriatr Psychiatry.*; 27(9):931-9. doi: 10.1002/gps.2804. Epub 2012 Mar 2.

24. Morris JC, Heymann A, Mohs RC, Hughes JP, van Belle G, Fillenbaum G, Mellits FD, Clark C. (1989). Consortium to establish a registry for Alzheimer disease (part 1) clinical and neuropsychological assessment. *Neurology, 39* (9) 1159-65.

25. Huppert FA, Byrane C, Gill C, Paykel ES, Beardsall L. (1995). CAMCOG. *Brit. J Clinc Psychol* 34)Pt 4) 529-41.

26. Agrell B, Delumn O. (1998). The Clock Drawing Test. *Age and Ageing* 27:399-403.

27. Folstein MF, Folstein SE, McHugh PR. (1975). Mini-mental state: a practical method for grading the cognitive state of patients for the clinician. *J Psychiatr Res.*; 12:189-198.

28. Baiyewu O, Unverzagt. FW , Lane KA, Gureje O, Muscik B, Gao S, Hall KS, Hendrie HC.(2005) Stick Design Test: A New Measure of

Visuoconstructional Ability. *Journal of International Neuropsychology Society.* 11: 598-605.

29. Paddick SM, Kisoli A, Longdon A, Dotchin C, Gray WK, Chaote P, Teodorczuk A, Walker R. (2015b). The prevalence and burden of behavioural and psychological symptoms of dementia in rural Tanzania. *Int J Geriatr Psychiatry.*; 30(8):815-23. doi: 10.1002/gps.4218. Epub 2014 Oct 28.

30. Paddick SM, Mkenda S, Mbowe G, Kisoli A, Gray WK, Dotchin CL, Ternent L, Ogunniyi A, Kissima J, Olakehinde O, Mushi D, Walker RW. (2017). Cognitive stimulation therapy as a sustainable intervention for dementia in sub-Saharan Africa: feasibility and clinical efficacy using a stepped-wedge design. *Int Psychogeriatr;* 29(6):979-989. doi: 10.1017/S1041610217000163. Epub 2017 Feb 22.

31. Adamis D, Ball C. (2000). Physical morbidity in elderly psychiatric inpatients: prevalence and possible relations between the major mental disorders and physical illness. *Int J Geriatr.*; 5(3):248-53.

32. Uwakwe R. (2000b). Psychiatric morbidity in elderly patients admitted to non-psychiatric wards in a general/teaching hospital in Nigeria. *Int J Geriatr Psychiatry;* 346-54.

33. Gureje O, Kola L, Afolabi E. (2007). Epidemiology of major depressive disorders in elderly Nigerians in Ibadan Study of Ageing: a community based study. *Lancet.* 15,370957-64.

34. Sokoya OO, Baiyewu O. (2003). Geriatric depression in Nigerian primary care attendees. *Int J Geriatr Psychiatry;* 18(6):506-10.

35. Baiyewu O, Yusuf AJ, Ogundele A. (2015). Depression in elderly people living in rural Nigeria and its association with perceived health, poverty, and social network. *Int Psychogeriatr;* 12):2009-15. doi0.1017/S1041610215001088. Epub 2015 Aug 12.

36. Olagunju AT, Olutoki MO, Ogunnubi OP, Adeyemi JD. (2015). Late-life depression: Burden, severity and relationship with social support dimensions in a West African community. *Arch Gerontol Geriatr;* 61(2):240-6. doi: 10.1016/j.archger.2015.05.002. Epub 2015 May.

37. Tomita A, Burns JK. (2013). Depression, disability and functional status among community-dwelling older adults in South Africa: evidence from the first South African National Income Dynamics Study. *Int J Geriatr Psychiatry;* 28(12):1270-9. doi: 10.1002/gps.3954. Epub 2013 Mar 20.

38. Ojagbemi A, Oladeji B, Abiona T, Gureje O. (2013). Suicidal behaviour in old age-results from the Ibadan Study of Ageing. *BMC Psychiatry.* 13;13:80. doi: 10.1186/1471-244X-13-80.

39. Lesher EL, Berryhill JS. (1994). Validation of the geriatric depression scale short form. *J Clin Psychol* 50: 256-260.

40. Maurer DM (2012) Screening for Depression. *Am Fam Physcian* 85(2) 139-144.

41. Pendlebury ST, Lovett NG, Smith SC, Dutta N, Bendon C, Lloyd-Lavery A, Mehta Z, Rothwell PM. (2015). Observational, longitudinal study of delirium in consecutive unselected acute medical admissions: age-specific rates and associated factors, mortality and re-admission. *BMJ Open* 2015;5:e00788. doi:10.1136.

42. Ola BA, Crabb J, Krishnadas R, Erinfolami AR, Olagunju A. (2010). Incidence and correlates of delirium in a West African mental health clinic. *Gen Hosp Psychiatry;* 32(2):176-81. doi: 10.1016/j.genhosppsych. 2009.10.005. Epub 2009 Nov 18.

43. Ojagbemi A, Owolabi M, Bello T, Baiyewu O. (2017). Stroke severity predicts poststroke delirium and its association with dementia: Longitudinal observation from a low income setting. *Journal of the Neurological Sciences* 375 : 376–381.

44. Caplan G. (2011) Managing Delirium in older patients. *Aust Prescr* 34: 16-18.

10

Culture and Mental Health

Olatunji F. Aina

Abstract

Mental health and culture are intertwined. Culture is a great determinant of mental well being and state of psychopathology. The symptomatic expression of virtually all psychiatric disorders is influenced by culture. Again, culture can be a causative factor of psychopathology, as obtained with culture bound syndromes. Despite the importance of culture in mental health, its appropriate consideration in psychiatric diagnosis and formulation was not to be until few years ago when the concept of cultural formulation came into being.

Culture also plays vital roles in perceived aetiologies and effective treatment of psychopathologies in various cultures. Particularly, in developing countries, supernatural and preternatural factors are largely believed to be the causes of mental illness. Thus, the pathway to care in such environs is tortuous, with the initial patronization of traditional healers before the mentally ill is taken to orthodox psychiatric facilities, only after treatment with traditional healers fail.

Another important issue in cultural psychiatry is migration. With migration, many mental health professionals nowadays practice in cultures alien to their own. Thus, there is emphasis now on cultural competence, that is acquisition of necessary skills to

> *manage the mentally-ill from different cultural*
> *backgrounds.*

Keywords: Mental health; inter-relationship culture and diagnosis; cultural competence; culture bound syndromes; migration and psychopathology.

Descriptions and definitions of culture

Culture is an important determinant of well-being, health and illness. It plays an important role in the shaping and modelling of individual and group behaviour in a defined society. Culture includes a number of variables such as traditions, religious beliefs, folklores, language, morals and values. In modern times, culture also includes financial philosophies and technological advances.

Tylor Edward[1] described culture as:

> . . . *that complex whole which includes knowledge,*
> *beliefs, art, morals, law, customs and any other*
> *capabilities and habits acquired by man as a*
> *member of society.*

In relation to mental health, culture is defined as:

> . . . *meanings, values and behavioural norms that*
> *are learned and transmitted in the dominant*
> *society and within its social groups. Thus, culture*
> *powerfully influences cognition, feelings and self-*
> *concept, as well as the diagnostic process and*
> *treatment decisions.*[2]

Culture and mental health are inter-twined and strongly related. Culture is an important determinant of the mental health of an individual or a group. Thus, mental illness is considered the product of a complex interaction of biological, psychological, social and cultural factors.

According to Pols,[3] the relationship between culture and mental health was first conceptualized by Emil Kraepilin. The mental health or well-being of an individual is described usually in reference to the culture or sub-cultural group he/she belongs. And the symptomatic manifestations of nearly all psychopathologies are coloured by the culture of the affected people. Thus, culture influences the cause, perception, symptomatology, course, health-seeking behaviour and treatment of mental illness.[4] Viswanath and Chaturvedi[5] regarded culture as that which strongly influences the phenomenology, epidemiology, treatment and outcome of mental illness.

Dimensions of transcultural psychiatry
Transcultural psychiatry deals with the socio-cultural aspects of human behaviour, mental health, psychiatric disorders and their treatment techniques. Transcultural psychiatry is described as the study of mental illness across various cultures, which includes its definitions, causality, classification and treatment in different cultural contexts. It is also known as cross-cultural psychiatry or ethno-psychiatry.

Nowadays among other issues, transcultural psychiatry deals with the following:
- Influence of culture on personality
- Cultural dynamics of migration and globalization

- Culture and psychopathology: psychiatric diagnosis, symptomatology, cross-cultural mental health assessment
- Treatment techniques in various cultural groups
- Ethno-psychopharmacology and folk medicine
- Culture and modern (western-oriented) health care services

Cross-cultural issues of mental health

What constitutes abnormal behaviour?

The social or cultural context in which behaviour occurs determines whether the behaviour is adjudged normal or abnormal. In the western world, major psychiatric illnesses, such as psychosis, minor mental illnesses (described by some as neuroses), personality disorders, eating disorders and so on are well-recognized. On the other hand, in developing countries, most especially in Africa, only persons with psychosis are usually recognized as mentally-ill. [6]

Causative factors of mental illness (MI)

In the Western world, mental illness are believed to be caused by scientific factors such as genetic inheritance, head injury, psychosocial trauma, etc; while in the developing world, such as in most of Asia and Africa, mental illness is generally believed to be supernatural. For instance, among the Maharashtrian culture in India, it is believed that being possessed by a spirit (*bhut bhada*) may give rise to trances, and more often results in ill health or bad luck. [5] In Africa, mental illness is believed to be the work of witches, demons, or as the result of some action that offended the gods or the ancestors.[4,7]

Health seeking behaviour and the treatment of mental illness

Culture influences, to a large extent, the health-seeking behaviour of persons with mental illness. Culture also influences the type of help they seek, and the type of coping styles and support they have. Consequently, acceptance and response to the various therapeutic modalities are influenced by culture. In any particular culture, healers and the healing practices used depend on the recognized aetiologies of mental illness. In developing countries, non-orthodox mental health care is largely utilized due to the perceived spiritual or preternatural causes of mental illness. As people believe in supernatural causation, they often approach traditional and spiritual faith healers for the treatment and to remove the causative evil agent.

In Africa, a wide variety of traditional healers are available to treat mental illness. Traditional healing involves the use of the following:

- Herbs
- Divination and incantations
- Offering of sacrifices
- Physical restraints (e.g., the use of shackles)
- Whips

Rehabilitation measures may also include home upkeep, running of errands, farming and 'gardening'.

Culture and psychopathology

For decades, biomedical explanations for psychiatric disorders held sway. However, in the past few years, the importance of socio-cultural factors in the aetio-pathogenesis of psychiatric disorders is being revisited. For instance, Marsella and Yamada[8] submitted that mental illness is firmly rooted in an individual's culture and other social factors. Different societal views about mental illness are strongly influenced by culture.

Tseng[9] asserted that culture has multiple roles to play in the expression of psychopathology. He gave the following seven types of clinical constructs of the cultural influence on psychopathology:

1. **Pathogenic effects:** Culture is a direct causative factor in forming or generating mental illness. Important examples here are the culture bound syndromes (CBS). The CBS, first coined by Yap,[10] are disorders that occur mainly in specific cultures or ethnic groups.

2. **Patho-selective effects:** This is the tendency to select culturally-influenced reactions to stress that shape the patterns of psychopathology.

3. **Patho-plastic effects:** Culture contributes to the modelling or shaping of the manifestations of psychopathology. That is, shaping the content of the symptoms, such as hallucinations, delusions, phobias or

obsessions is subject to psychosocial context in which the pathology is reported.

4. **Patho-elaborating effect**: Certain behaviours become exaggerated sometimes even to the extreme through cultural reinforcements.

5. **Patho-facilitative effects**: Psychological and socio-cultural factors contribute to the occurrence of many psychiatric disorders, for example, alcohol and substance use disorders.

6. **Patho-reactive effects**: Culture influences perception and reaction, that is, how people label a disorder and how they emotionally react to it.

7. **Patho-discriminative effects**: Culture influences the socio-culturally labelling of behaviour as normal or abnormal. For instance, personality disorders and substance abuse are either accepted or rejected in a society according to the prevailing cultural factors.

Generally, the inter-relationship between culture and psychopathologies is captured in two schools of thought:

The universalistic school

The main thrust here is that the basic psychopathology of all mental disorders is universal and that cross-cultural differences in clinical patterns derive mainly from culture-specific illness behaviour. In other words, culture is pathoplastic. This universalistic school is also known as the etic school. According to the universalistic school, the underlying cultural processes are the same across cultures all over the world. That is, psychological distress is experienced all over the world, but culture modifies its expression. Thus, nosological diagnostic entities developed in western countries are applicable to other cultures.

The relativistic (emic) school

The philosophy in this school is that a full aetiological understanding of many psycho-pathologies depends largely on cultural factors. Furthermore, according to this school, there are a number of disorders which have been found to be culture-specific, and in which cultural factors have been demonstrated to play a major aetiological role, that is, the so-called culture-bound syndromes (CBS).

In other words, culture can also be pathogenic. Some examples of CBS include: Koro, Amok, Brain Fag, Shen kui, Zar, Dhat, etc. However, research has not yet determined whether culture-bound syndromes are distinct from established mental disorders, or are variants of them. Furthermore, a number of CBS or culture-related problems which have been described in many developing countries (particularly in Africa) are not listed in the current classification systems of mental disorders.[7]

Culture in psychiatric diagnosis

Psychiatric diagnosis entails making appropriate clinical deductions following a thorough clinical evaluation and assessment of a patient. In the practice of psychiatry, diagnosis employs the syndromic approach, in contrast to aetiological diagnoses in other medical specialties.

The symptomatic manifestations of nearly all psycho-pathologies are coloured by the culture of the affected people. Culture can also be a trigger of psychiatric illness. Thus, cultural factors are important in psychiatric diagnosis.[7] However, in modern psychiatric practice, the perception of culture as a considerable factor in psychiatric assessment and diagnosis is still very limited. At best, there is only a mention of cultural factors such as race, language, ethnicity— particularly the minorities and migrant status—when culture is even considered by mental health professionals.

Aside from what obtains in clinical practice, the internationally-accepted psychiatric diagnostic systems did not give due recognition to culture until the modest recognition accorded to it in the fourth edition of the diagnostic and statistical manual (DSM-IV) by the American Psychiatric Association (APA), where there is an inclusion of a cultural formulation in the appendix and a glossary of culture-bound syndromes. The latest version of the diagnostic and statistical manual (DSM-V) gives a more remarkable recognition to culture in psychiatric diagnosis.[11] For instance, the concept of culture-bound syndromes in DSM-IV has been replaced by an expanded description in DSM-V within the following three concepts:

- Cultural syndromes
- Cultural idioms of distress
- Cultural explanations of distress or perceived causes

It is also envisioned that subsequent versions of DSM would be progressively more inclusive of psychopathologies across various cultures of the world.[11,12]

In the international classification of diseases (ICD) by World Health Organization (WHO), the cultural component of psychiatric diagnosis is yet to be given due recognition even in the current 10th edition (ICD-10). It is hoped that ICD-11, already in the pipeline, would address these issues.

Cultural formulation

The importance of culture in mental health care has taken a formidable position more so with the incorporation of cultural considerations into clinical assessment and diagnostic formulation in the past few decades. The American Psychiatric Association (APA) particularly drives the concept of cultural formulation through its incorporation into the DSM system.

> *The cultural formulation provides a systematic review of the individual's cultural background, the role of the cultural context in the expression and evaluation of symptoms and dysfunction.*[13]

The idea of cultural formulation was mooted in the course of preparing DSM-III, but became crystallized and incorporated into DSM-IV. The main goal of cultural formulation is to assist clinicians in identifying cultural-contextual factors that can potentially affect the patient in the therapeutic setting.

The cultural formulation interview (CFI) is a new innovation in DSM-V. It produces the DSM-IV outline for cultural formulation (OCF) into a set of questions and explicit instructions. The outline for cultural formulation comprises the following:

- Cultural identity of the person
- Cultural explanations of individual's illness
- Cultural factors related to psychosocial environment and levels of functioning
- Cultural elements of the relationship between the individual and the clinician
- Overall cultural assessment regarding diagnosis and care

Cultural competence

Culture plays a vital role in an individual's health and state of illness. Due to migration, many clinicians nowadays practice in countries or environments different from their own culture. Thus, there is the need for them to understand the culture of their clients to be able to establish a good therapeutic alliance. Therefore, the concept of cultural competence (CC) entails the ability of health professionals to interact effectively with patients or clients of different ethnic or cultural backgrounds.

According to Cross:[14]

> . . . *cultural competence is a set of congruent behaviours, attitudes and policies that come together in a system, an agency or among*

> *professionals that enables them to work effectively*
> *in cross-cultural situations.*

A more recent definition given to CC by the Joint Commission on Culture and Psychiatry(2010),[15] which conveys essentially the same meaning as that given above, goes thus:

> *Cultural competence (CC) is the ability of health*
> *care providers and health care organizations to*
> *understand and respond effectively to the cultural*
> *and language needs brought by the patient to the*
> *health care encounter.*

Components of cultural competence
According to Papadopoulous,[16] the essential components of cultural competence include the following:

1. **Cultural desire**: Motivation to acquire cross-cultural knowledge for the development of cultural competence.

2. **Cultural awareness**: Knowledge of cultural understanding of self to avoid conflicts and bias.

3. **Attitude**: Practitioner's attitudinal disposition to cultural diversity.

4. **Knowledge of diverse cultural practices and world views**: This involves the acquisition of cross-cultural knowledge to enhance practice in a cultural diverse setting.

5. **Cross-cultural skills**: Competency in cross-cultural practice

Migration, culture and mental illness

Migration, a stressful life event, can influence mental health. The world is now a global village with people of different cultural backgrounds relocating to various parts of the world for different reasons, such as to seek better economic opportunities or asylum, and due to displacement from war zones among others. A number of potential mental health issues associated with migration, among many other problems, include the following:

- Problems of communication, such as difficulty with one's accent and with understanding the foreign language.

- Difficulty in educational pursuit of the emigrants and their children.

- Experience of discrimination and cultural prejudice

- Experience of cultural shock

- Cultural conflicts of the clinicians practising in a foreign land and culture

- Increased vulnerability to mental illnesses, such as adjustment disorder, delusional disorder, depression, etc.

- Acculturation: This occurs during the process of adapting to a new culture. Berry[17] described acculturation as the cultural change that takes place when two different cultural groups come in contact. In other words, the acculturation process is at group level. However, acculturation change can also affect the migrant's identity and status at the individual level.

Culture and psychiatric stigma

Stigma for mental illness is universal, but there are cultural variations in the extent and type of stigma displayed for mental illness. Stigma tends to be more in the developing countries of the world.[18,19]

There are many definitions of stigma, such as

> . . . *a mark of disgrace associated with a particular circumstance, quality or person*

> . . . a *degrading and debasing attitude of the society that discredits a person or a group because of an attribute such as illness, deformity, colour, religion, nationality, etc.*

Mental illness constitutes 11% of the global burden of diseases. Three out of four (75%) people with mental illness report that they have experienced stigma. Stigma against people with mental illness involves inaccurate and hurtful representations of them as violent, comical or incompetent, thereby dehumanizing them and making them objects of fear or ridicule.

Conclusion

Culture and mental health are intertwined. Culture is an important determinant of mental health and state of illness.

Culture influences health-seeking behaviour and the types of treatment taken. In mental health, culture matters.

Learning points and objectives

- Understand the concept of culture and its inter-relationship with mental health.
- The role of culture in psychiatric diagnosis and management.
- Understand the concepts of cultural formulation and cultural competence in current mental health practice.
- Inter-relationship between migration and mental health.
- The influence of culture on psychiatric stigma.

References

1. Tylor EB. *Anthropology: an Introduction to the Study of Man and Civilization.* Macmillan and Co., London, 1871.
2. Mezzich. JE. *Culture and Psychiatric Diagnosis. A DSM-IV Perspective.* American Psychiatric Association Publishing, Arlington, VA, 2002.
3. Pols H.. Emil Kraepelin on cultural and ethnic factors in mental illness. *Psychiatric Times* 2011; 28(8): 1-6.
4. Aina OF. (2006). Psychotherapy by environment manipulation and the observed symbolic rites on prayer mountains in Nigeria. *Mental Health, Religion and Culture* 2; 9(1):1-13.
5. Viswanath B, Chaturvedi SK. Cultural aspects of major mental disorders: A critical review from an Indian perspective. *Indian Journal of Psychological Medicine* 2012; 34(4): 306-312.
6. Aina OF, Famuyiwa OO. Ogun–Oru: A traditional explanation for nocturnal neuropsychiatric disturbances among the Yoruba of south west Nigeria. *Transcultural Psychiatry* 2007; 44: 44- 54.

7.   Aina OF, Morakinyo O. Culture-bound syndromes and the neglect of cultural factors in psychopathologies among Africans. *African Journal of Psychiatry* 2011; 14: 278-285.

8.   Marsella AJ, Yamada AM. Culture and mental health: An introduction and overview of foundations, concepts and issues, p. 3-24. In: I. Cuellar, F. Paniagua, editors. *Handbook of Multicultural Mental Health*. Academic Press, New York, 2000.

9.   Tseng W. (2001). Culture and psychopathology. In: S. Diego, editor. *Handbook of Cultural Psychiatry*. Academic Press, CA, USA, 2001.

10. Yap PM. The culture bound syndromes, p. 33-53. In: W. Cahil, TY Lin, Editos. *Mental Health Research in Asia and the Pacific*. East-West Centre Press, Honolulu, 1969.

11. Lewis-Fernández R, Aggarwal NK, Bäärnhielm S, Rohlof H, Kirmayer LJ, Weiss MG, Jadhav S, Hinton L, Alarcón RD, Bhugra D, Groen S, van Djik R, Qureshi A, Collazos F, Rousseau C, Caballero L, Ramos M, Lu F. Culture and psychiatric evaluation: Operationalizing cultural formulation for DSM-5. *Psychiatry* 2014; 77(2):130-154.

12. Parnas J, Gallagher S. Phenomenology and the interpretation of psychopatological experience. In: L. Kirmayer, R. Lemelson, C. Cummings, editors. *Revisioning Psychiatry Integrating*. Cambridge University Press, Cambridge, 2015.

13. American Psychiatric Association. *Diagnostic and Statistical Manual (DSM) of Mental Disorders*. 4th edition. American Psychological Association, Washington DC, 2000.

14. Cross TL, Bazron BJ, Dennis KW, Isaacs MR. Towards a culturally competent system of care. A monograph on effective services for minority children who are severely emotionally disturbed. National Criminal Justice Reference Service. http://www.ncjrs.gov/App/ Publications/abstract.aspx?ID=124939 (Accessed on 18 March 2017).

15. The Joint Commission: *Advancing Effective Communication, Cultural Competence, and Patient- and Family-Centered Care: A Roadmap for Hospitals*. The Joint Commission, 2010.

16. Papadopoulous RK. Trauma in a systematic perspective: Theoretical, organizational and clinical dimensions. Paper presented at the 2004 XIV congress of the International Family Therapy Association, Istanbul, Turkey.

17. Berry JW, Kim U, Minde T, Mok D. (1987). Comparative studies of acculturative stress. *International Migration Review* 1987; 21: 491-511.

18. Sussman LK. The use of herbal preventive treatment for pregnant women and neonates among the Mahafaly of southern Madagascar. Annual Meeting of American Anthropological Association, 1988.

19. Wahl OF. Mental health consumer's experience of stigma. *Schizophrenia Bulletin* 1999; 25(3): 467-478.

Selected readings

Mezzich JE, Kleimman A, Fabrega H, Parron DL. *Culture and Psychiatric Diagnoses. A DSM-IV Perspective.* American Psychiatric Press, Washington DC; London, England, 2005, p. xvii-14.

Pandey, J. Psychology in India enters the twenty-first century: Movement toward an indigenous discipline, p. 342–366. In J. Pandey, editor. *Psychology in India Revisited: Developments in the Discipline.* Vol. 3. SAGE Publications, New Delhi, 2004.

Sam DL, Moreira V. Revisiting the mutual embeddedness of culture and mental Illness. *Online Readings in Psychology and Culture* 2012; 10(2).

Subudi C. Culture and mental illness. *Social Work Practice in Mental Health: Cross-Cultural Perspectives* 2015; 132-140.

Yap PM. Words and things in comparative psychiatry with special reference to the exotic psychoses. *Acta Psychiatrica Scandinavica* 1962; 38: 163-169.

11

Interface between Historical Group Trauma and Contemporary Politics in Nigeria: The Civil War Experience

Femi Adebajo

Historical evolution of diagnostic concepts

It has long been recognized that traumatic events can lead to psychological consequences in individuals and whole communities. The modern understanding of the clinical aspects of trauma sequelae and their codification into reproducible categories began after the First World War. Prior to this, it had been thought that the development of severe and sustained psychological problems after a traumatic event was indicative of abnormal personality traits and an underlying neurosis, since transient and self-limiting reactions were held to be the norm.[1,2]

The modern understanding of the psychological responses to traumatic events in western psychiatry was influenced by the experiences of combat veterans in the First World War. This has led to an increasing recognition that certain stressful events directly lead to psychological symptoms in some individuals. The codification of these symptom clusters into diagnostic categories as an aid to clinical practice and research, began with the inclusion of post-traumatic stress disorder (PTSD) as a diagnostic category in the third edition of the Diagnostic and Statistical Manual (DSM-III)[3] and the further elaboration of the diagnostic criteria, symptom classification and duration, and clinical description in DSM-IIIR and the International Classification of Diseases-Version 10 (ICD-10).[4] The operational definitions had been further refined in the later editions of DSM and DCR to account for findings from recent epidemiological research evidence.

Clinical features

- *Acute stress reaction:* Dissociative symptoms (depersonalization, derealization, amnesia, emotional numbing, reduced feeling)
- *PTSD*: Delayed/protracted reaction, traumatic stressors — life-threatening and/or catastrophic (death/severe injury/threat to physical integrity)
- *Three symptom clusters*: Re-experiencing, avoidance and hyperarousal

DSM-V/IV and ICD-10 criteria

1. **Stressor criterion**
   - Event or situation of exceptionally threatening or catastrophic nature
   - Likely to cause pervasive distress to almost anyone

2. **Symptom criteria**
   - Repetitive intrusive recollection or re-enactment of the event in memories, daytime imagery or dreams

- Sense of numbness or emotional blunting, detachment from others, unresponsiveness to surroundings, anhedonia
- Avoidance of activities and situations reminiscent of trauma
- Autonomic hyperarousal with hypervigilance, enhanced startle reaction, insomnia
- Anxiety and depression
- Dramatic bursts of fear, panic or aggression triggered by reminders

3. **Duration criteria**

- Symptoms usually arise within 6 months of the traumatic event

4. **Disability criteria**

- Clinically significant distress or impairment in social, occupational or other important areas of functioning
- This criteria is required in DSM-IV, but not in ICD-10.

Pathophysiological mechanisms

Hypothalamic-pituitary-adrenal axis abnormalities

- Enhanced negative feedback and large responses to further stressors
- Reduced basal cortisol levels in PTSD patients compared with normal controls and traumatized minus PTSD

- Increased number of lymphocyte glucocorticoid receptors
- Enhanced response on dexamethasone suppression test

Neuroendocrine abnormalities

- Dysregulation of several neurotransmitter systems
- Down-regulation of alpha2-adrenergic receptors
- Enhanced activity in locus coeruleus
- Increased levels of noradrenaline — autonomic hyperarousal
- Sensitized serotonergic system
- Conditioned secretion of endorphins and analgesia when exposed to reminders of trauma
- Enhanced levels of corticotrophin-releasing factor
- Dopamine, GABA and N-methyl-p-aspartate systems

Thyroid

- Increased thyroid hormones in some patients, correlated with severity of hyperarousal symptoms

Neuroimaging
MRI

- Reduced hippocampal volumes in veterans and women with history of childhood sexual abuse (CSA)
- Animal studies show association between high cortisol levels during stress and hippocampal damage

PET studies

- Relative reduction in middle temporal flow (and adjacent middle frontal areas); the mPFC plays a role in the extinction of fear by the inhibition of the amygdala function
- PTSD patients show increased blood flow in limbic regions (parahippocampus and cingulate)

Differential diagnosis

Diagnostic hierarchy is usually suspended. Hence, co-morbidity is common. About 80% of PTSD patients have other psychiatric diagnoses. Epidemiological surveys indicate that the most common co-morbid conditions are depressive disorders, substance misuse disorders and anxiety disorders.[5] Attempts to explain this phenomenon have included hypotheses about the symptom overlaps in the relevant diagnostic categories, under-diagnosis of PTSD, especially where trauma history is not specifically sought, self-medication with illicit drugs and alcohol, and the exaggeration of symptoms by withdrawal phenomena. Differentiation can be made with careful history-taking to establish differences in symptom duration, symptom severity, symptom clusters, stressor characteristics and associated functional impairment.

Acute stress reaction

- Adjustment disorders
- Acute polymorphic psychotic disorder
- Dissociative disorders
- Depersonalization (derealization syndrome)

- Enduring personality change after a catastrophic experience

Trauma in large populations

A whole range of traumatic events and disasters are a part of modern human experience, ranging from wars, political violence, civil disturbances, large-scale accidents and natural disasters. The effects of these disasters on the human psyche are modulated by the feelings, thoughts and behaviours that are inevitable human responses to such seismic events. Thankfully, such emotional reactions are short-lived in most individuals, but there is a significant minority in whom the emotional sequelae of disasters persist long after the traumatic events have ended.

Each individual experiences and responds to trauma in a unique way that is influenced by how much meaning they attach to the event in question, itself a derivative of the person's make up and the social context in which the individual exists. The subsequent manifestation of post-traumatic sequelae and individual adjustment is influenced by both individual and group psychology. Psychological themes applicable to the individual include individual cognitive style, personal meaning, loss of autonomy and control, as well as perceptions of vulnerability, finding a meaning ("why me?") and susceptibility to the loss of personal physical and emotional security.

The relevant group mechanisms include family bonds, communal support mechanisms, cultural norms, beliefs and practices that exert a powerful normative influence on individual responses. In particular, the heterogeneity of the group norms may explain the observable differences in group responses to similar traumatic events. For example, the low rates of PTSD observed in the survivors of the civil wars in Sierra Leone and Liberia in the 1990s.[6,7] It is unclear if the lower than expected PTSD rates indicate a true difference in incidence, or is an artifact of under-reporting or low research interest and health provision, but the role of age at exposure, gender and levels of post-conflict community acceptance, as protective factors, have been studied by specific cohort studies. This is an area for further research.

Ethnic riots and vicarious trauma

According to Donald Horowitz, "deadly ethnic riot is an intense, though not necessarily wholly unplanned, lethal attack by civilian members of one ethnic group on civilian members of another ethnic group, the victims chosen because of their group membership."[8] The 1966 anti-Igbo pogrom in Northern Nigeria is a classic example of this form of collective violence. The morphology and dynamics of the violence makes it possible to identify patterns in precipitants, targets, supporting conditions, location and riot behaviour, that offer an insight into both the immediate traumatogenic effects and propensity for long-term re-experiencing of the trauma. In particular, both selective targeting and randomness did occur in various individuals, leading to further heterogeneity of subjective experience.

Nigerian Civil War experience

The Nigerian Civil War, also known as the Nigeria-Biafra War, was the first large-scale military conflict in post-colonial

Africa, and it lasted for 925 days. It was preceded, between 1962 and 1966, by civilian ethnicity-based pogroms, large-scale riots, political unrest and violence. The exact figures of human casualties are disputed, but most reasonable estimates place them near the 2 million mark. It is therefore reasonable to estimate the number of people exposed to traumatogenic events in the tens of millions, including victims, perpetrators and observers.

Politically-driven violence tends to be unpredictable, random and a cause great fear, and the events of the 1962-1966 period in Nigeria were no different. Various communal disturbances took a violent turn and this in turn attracted repressive countermeasures from government law enforcement agents. All of these events inevitably involve the use of violence against persons, with attendant physical and mental injury. The 1962-70 epoch is very well-documented in books, films and oral accounts, and there is no doubt that the whole range of traumatogenic circumstances (famine, starvation, dislocation, loss of property, imprisonment, physical injury, mutilation, rape, explosions, genocide, violent deaths) were experienced by a large number of people.

Social and political aspects
The fractious nature of Nigeria's peculiar identity and ethnic politics has meant that the civil unrest in the First Republic leading to the military interventions in 1966, have continued to play a large role in subsequent decades. A lack of clear vision about the mechanisms of reconciliation and individual accounting has led to an uncoordinated series of individualized responses to the traumas of this turbulent

period. Many victims have simply elected to get on with life, as best as they can, while relegating their experiences to the recesses of their private thoughts. Others have written accounts of their experiences, variously as historical narratives, cathartic exercises and exculpatory efforts. The net result is a cacophony of accounts, discordant, angry and sometimes venomous contentions that have hung over individual and group relations within the country ever since the formal end of the war in 1970. The official attempts at reconciliation have been interpreted as generous by some, insincere and tokenistic by others. A perception of continuing official persecution and punishment exists very strongly in the communities that suffered the greatest privations of the war era.

On the individual level, it does not appear that a coherent strategy existed to determine the extent of post-traumatic sequelae in various Nigerian sub-populations and, informal mechanisms, based within families and self-help efforts of communities, have been the only solution to this problem. There are numerous anecdotes of people 'not being the same' after the war, but it seems this is ever acknowledged as treatable psychological morbidity. There is hardly any epidemiological data on the prevalence of mental disorders after the Nigerian Civil War, and most of the commentary has alluded to projections from other African conflict zones.[9,10]

Healing the wounds

A holistic approach is required to manage this complex series of difficulties, drawing on communal mechanisms, including religious beliefs and cultural norms, as well as the recognition and treatment of specific disorders in individuals. The use of recognized treatments, mainly SSRI antidepressants for PTSD, as well as trauma-focussed cognitive behavioural therapy (CBT) adapted to local circumstances. The opportunity for catharsis should be grasped by a careful negotiation of the desire to forget on the part of victims and perpetrators alike, and the likelihood of denial, blame shifting and defensive justification of atrocities. Genuine national reconciliation effort, drawing on the recent experiences of Rwanda and South Africa, possibly combined with a rigorous academic documentation of history, would be important for group healing and the prevention of future disturbances.[1,2]

References

1. Van der Kolk BA, Weisaeth L, Van der Hart O. History of trauma in psychiatry, p. 47-74. In BA Van der Kolk, AC McFarlane, L Weisaeth (Eds) *Traumatic Stress*. Guildford Press, New York, 1996.

2. Gersons BPR, Carlier IVE. Post-traumatic stress disorder: The history of a recent concept. *British Journal of Psychiatry* 1992; 161: 742-8.

3. American Psychiatric Association. *Diagnostic and Statistical Manual* (DSM-III). 3rd edition. American Psychiatric Association, Washington DC, 1980.

4. WHO. *The ICD-10 Classification of Mental and Behavioural Disorders: Clinical Descriptions and Diagnostic Guidelines*. World Health Organization, Geneva. 1992

5. Brady KT, Killeen TK, Brewerton T, Lucerini S. Comorbidity of psychiatric disorders and posttraumatic stress disorder. *J Clin Psychiatry*, 2010; 17: 22-32

6. Betancourt TS, Newnham EA, McBain R, Brennan RT. Post-traumatic stress symptoms among former child soldiers in Sierra Leone: Follow-

up study. *The British Journal of Psychiatry* 2013; 203(3):196-202. doi:10.1192/bjp.bp.112.113514.

7.   Betancourt TS, Borisova II, Williams TP, Brennan RT, Whitfield TH, De La Soudiere M, Williamson J, Gilman SE. Sierra Leone's former child soldiers: A follow-up study of psychosocial adjustment and community reintegration. *Child Development* 2010; 81(4):1077-95.

8.   Horowitz DL. *The Deadly Ethnic Riot.* University of California Press, Berkeley, Los Angeles, 2001.

9.   Njenga FG, Nguithi AN, Kang'ethe RN. War and mental disorders in Africa. *World Psychiatry* 2006; 5(1):38-39.

10. Atwoli L, Stein DJ, Williams DR, Mclaughlin KA, Petukhova M, Kessler RC, Koenen KC. (2013). Trauma and posttraumatic stress disorder in South Africa: Analysis from the South African Stress and Health Study. *BMC Psychiatry* 2013; 13: 182.

Selected readings

American Psychiatric Association. *Diagnostic and Statistical Manual of Mental Disorders: DSM-IV-TR.* American Psychiatric Association, Washington DC, 2000.

American Psychiatric Association. *Diagnostic and Statistical Manual of Mental Disorders: DMSV-5-TR.* American Psychiatric Association, ashington DC, 2013.

Gelder MG, Lopez-Ibor JJ, Andreasen NC. *New Oxford Textbook of Psychiatry.* Vol. 1. Oxford University Press, Oxford, 2000.

Gould M. *the Biafran War: the struggle for modern Nigeria.* IB Tauris, New York:, 2013.

Johnstone EC, Owens DC, Lawrie SM. *Companion to Psychiatric Studies.* 7th ed. Elsevier Health Sciences, Amsterdam, 2010.

Ursano RJ, Fullerton CS, McCaughey BG. *Trauma and Disaster,* p. 3-27. In RJ Ursano, BG McCaughey, CS Fullerton, editors. *Individual and Community Responses to Trauma and Disaster: the structure of human chaos.* University Press, Cambridge, 1994.

12

Mental Health Legislation in sub-Saharan Africa

Jibril Abdulmalik, Adegboyega Ogunwale &
Akintunde Akinkunmi

Abstract

The global mental health efforts to improve mental health services delivery in low and middle income countries, including sub-Saharan African countries, are unlikely to yield dividends without an enabling policy and legislative framework. Mental health legislation should guarantee the rights and protection of persons with mental disorders.

Many SSA countries do not have a stand-alone mental health legislation, as just over half (55%) are reported to have one. The majority of these countries with mental health legislation have obsolete and stigmatizing content that were inherited, in most cases, from the colonial era. Many SSA countries currently do not have any mental health legislation. It is therefore imperative to encourage the revision of outdated laws in SSA, as well as the passage of such updated versions where they exist, such as in Nigeria and Uganda.

However, South Africa (in 2002) and Ghana more recently (2012) have updated their mental health legislation in line with global best practices and are utilizing a rights-based approach. The process is usually an arduous task but persistent advocacy and perseverance is crucial for success.

Keywords: Mental health legislation; sub-Saharan Africa

233

Introduction

The poor state of mental health services delivery in sub-Saharan Africa (SSA) is not only due to the pervasive and age-old problems of insufficient resources and under-funding but also largely due to a poor regulatory framework — in terms of mental health policies and legislation. Mental health policies essentially provide a vision and an outline of a country's commitment to the mental health needs of her people. But the recommendations of a policy document are merely advisory and would necessarily require legal backing in the form of mental health legislation. This is especially true in SSA where widespread stigma, ignorance and human rights abuses against persons with mental disorders are rife.

A round table conference of leading mental health professionals on the African continent recently held in Stellenbosch, South Africa concluded that

> . . . *It is necessary for governments to have a robust legislative response to counter inhumane practices against those who are suffering, such as institutionalization, imprisonment, isolation, discrimination in access to public goods, and other violations of their human rights.*[1]

Mental health legislation remains a veritable tool for the protection, improvement and promotion of the mental well-being of citizens in countries across the world.[2] It further provides an enabling environment for the strengthening and enforcement of the fundamental human rights of those who suffer from mental disorders. Indeed, a number of human rights declarations, conventions and principles including the Universal Declaration of Human Rights[3], Principles for the Protection of Persons with Mental Illness[4], European Convention on Human Rights[5] and the African Charter on Human and People's Rights[6], among others have fuelled a rights-based approach to the enactment of mental health laws.

This approach has strongly influenced the global view at the level of the World Health Organization (WHO) on what constitutes meaningful and contemporary legislation.[2] While it may be argued that general or common law ought to be sufficient in dealing with the care of persons with mental disorders, experience and history suggest that dedicated mental health legislation will more adequately take their rights into consideration.[7]

The latest WHO Mental Health Atlas estimates that just over half (55%) of the countries in SSA currently have any mental health legislation.[8] This is in stark contrast to Europe where 91.8% of the countries have mental health legislation. A critical evaluation of this figure alarmingly reveals that some of these laws in SSA countries date back to the colonial era of the early 1900s.[9,10] In the absence of contemporary and rights-based mental health legislation in SSA, it is to be expected that the rights of person with mental disorders will be trampled upon and disrespected under the guise of beneficent paternalism which has been the default mode of many African societies in dealing with people with mental disorders. This chapter focuses on the evolution and current status of illustrative mental health legislation in selected countries in sub-Saharan Africa.

Ghana

Ghana passed a revised Mental Health Act in 2012[11] after several years of advocacy and concerted efforts by the mental health community, with support from Basic Needs Ghana, the Ministry of Health as well as the World Health Organization which provided technical support and input. The MHA (2012) aims to enhance access to mental health care services in the least restrictive environment, while encouraging early identification and prompt treatment of mental disorders within the primary care system. It also extends oversight functioning over private and public facilities as well as unorthodox facilities that provide services for persons with mental disorders. It emphasizes a rights-based approach that is in line with current evidence and best global practices.

Similar to what has occurred, and continues to happen in most SSA countries, it took several decades before this revision finally came to fruition. Historically, the first Ghanaian mental health legislation was the Lunatic Asylum Ordinance, Cap 79 of 1888, which laid the foundation for the establishment of the first asylum in 1906. This was minimally revised and passed as the Mental Health Act of 1972, which remained in force until the recently passed Mental Health Act of 2012.[12]

The MHA (2012) enables the establishment of a Mental Health Authority Board, which will provide oversight for the implementation of quality mental health care services in compliance with the MHA. However, the funding mechanisms for this authority are yet to be specified and are dependent on the eventual passage of the Legislative Instrument (LI) for them to be specified. The MHA enshrines the rights of persons with mental disorders, as well as protects against acts of discrimination in everyday life and employment. It also clearly stipulates the guidelines for voluntary and involuntary admissions; and the protection of vulnerable groups such as women, children, the elderly, and persons with intellectual disabilities.[13]

Some of the anticipated challenges with the implementation of the MHA, which were subsequently affirmed by a qualitative study with experienced key informants, were the need for training and improved expertise within the mental health system, the judiciary as well as social services; in addition to funding require-ments.[14,15] The most pertinent barrier, thus far, is the slow pace of the parliamentary process required to ensure the passage of the LI. This final step is crucial to enable the mobilization of resources for the implementation of the MHA.

The immediate next steps and focus for advocacy should include widespread public enlightenment campaigns, ensuring the passage of the LI, empowering the Mental Health Authority Board through the release of funds, improving the number of skilled mental health personnel as well as strengthening the legal infrastructure for the optimal performance of the mental health review tribunals. Furthermore, there is a need to revise other Ghanaian legislation such as the Criminal Code of Ghana and the Persons with Disability Act of Ghana, as they still classify attempted suicide as a criminal offence.[13]

Nigeria

Mental health legislation in Nigeria dates back to 1916,[16] which was over four decades before the country attained independence from British colonial rule. At commencement, it had the status of an ordinance but gradually became the framework for regional laws as the country progressed into distinct regions. It attained the status of a law in 1959 with its clearly colonial orientation intact since commencement. As the regions became disaggregated into distinct federating states, the lunacy law became state laws within the federation with each of the 36 states of the federation having its own lunacy law largely reminiscent of the ordinance of 1916 (for example, *Laws of Ogun State, 2006*).

While these state laws have attempted minor alterations in relation to language and certain provisions (for example the size of fines) in order to take cognizance of existent realities, it is instructive to note that the current laws retain the derogatory term of 'lunacy' for titular and practical purposes despite the obsolete nature of such a view of mental disorders. With mental health legislation being slightly over a century old in Nigeria at the moment, four critical areas have been identified in previous research as being largely responsible for the archaic nature of the law, namely:

   i.   Socio-political evolution in the country

ii.   Antiquated terminology

iii.   Apparent insulation from later and recent developments in psychopharmacology

iv.   As well as growing alternatives to custodial care and non-application of human rights.[17]

A critical review of the current law using the WHO guidelines for mental legislation[2] shows that the law lacks a focus on human rights and non-discrimination, access to services and least restrictive treatment alternatives. Its definitions are largely inadequate in terms of humaneness and scope. It continues to employ denigrating terms such as 'lunatic', 'idiot' and 'unsound' mind while focusing almost entirely on custodial care. It fails to define 'mental disorder' or 'mental disability' and has no clear posture towards dissocial personality, psychopathy or substance use disorders as important considerations in the elucidation of mental disorders from a psycho-legal point of view.

The current law has been unable to adequately provide for mental health care on an equal footing with physical health, and gives no attention to mental health care financing or access to such services within primary care settings even though it envisages the presence of 'asylums' which would usually be established by 'local government councils' (ss. 1–3). This may perhaps suggest that an attempt was being made to provide some expansion of access to custodial services.

While the law indirectly suggests that persons with mental disorders should not be unduly victimized within asylums, it fails to focus clearly on such rights as those related to dignity and human autonomy and provides no direction as to healthcare issues such as consent, privacy as well as confidentiality. It makes no mention of the rights of families or care givers of persons with mental disorders in relation to the right to information at and during an admission, the right to appeal involuntary admission, etc. Voluntary admission and treatment approaches to dealing with the non-protesting/incompetent patient as well as core capacity issues are not addressed in any meaningful way. Again, this may not be unexpected in the rather paternalistic context of colonialism and African communitarianism in which the law was crafted and continues to operate.

A most critical lapse in the law is that it does not specify the criteria of potential harm to self or others as a core basis for involuntary admission. Rather, it places this ground in the realm of apparent 'suspicion of lunacy' of mind, which renders the individual a suitable candidate for confinement. It also does not separate involuntary admission and treatment, thereby suggesting that admission is a prima facie basis for treatment without any emphasis on the competency of the patient to consent or withhold consent to treatment. This is also not extremely surprising given the fact that a global shift towards explicit consent of individuals began post-World War II with the adoption of the Nuremberg Code[18] and further contributions from the medical community.[19]

However, it is impressive to note that as early as the 1916 law, a reasonable attempt had been made to establish clear provisions for patients' involuntary admission on an emergency basis for a period not exceeding seven days (section 10). Evidently, while the more libertarian and individualistic view of rights as espoused in the present day would suggest that a more normative duration be markedly less than seven days[2], the presence of a defined duration and some level of criteria determination for emergency admission are still supportive of human dignity and autonomy.

The oversight and review mechanisms under the law are rather weak because they only relate to the establishment of a 3-man 'visiting committee' to asylums (ss. 7-9). This committee is expected to visit the facilities once a year, review 'complaints' and revert to the governor. Clearly, this arrangement does not provide clear directions on appeals, and even if a patient did complain, it might have been left unattended for about a year. While the law does not provide specific police duties as expected, it indicates that 'any person' can assist in returning an escapee lunatic back to an asylum. This broad interpretation of 'any person' may thus apply to the police as well. The current law is completely silent on special treatments, seclusion and restraints as well as clinical experimentation and research, discrimination, civil issues, housing, employment, social security and protection of vulnerable groups.

In view of the severe deficiencies of the current legislation, several attempts have been made to enact a brand new national mental health act, which will apply in all states of the federation. The most recent attempts started in 1999 during the fourth republic. While it appeared that the push gained momentum because the bill scaled through the first of three readings, the draft legislation suffered a set-back with the expiry of that senate and the death of the lead sponsor.[17] Several versions of the bill have been made since 2003 and the most current one appears to be the 2013 bill, which has attempted to address many of the lapses observed until then. It remains to be seen how this bill will fare in the corridors of legislation at the national level. However, it is interesting to note that in the last few years, an attempt has been made to seek a state-based mental health 'law' in Lagos State of Nigeria (the most advanced state in the country) rather than an act of the National Assembly. This appears more consistent with the natural history of mental health legislation in Nigeria. That said, the draft bill for the mental health law is currently between the executive and legislative arms of government.

South Africa

South Africa (and Ghana) currently boasts of the most advanced mental health legislation that is in tandem with global best practices in SSA. The Mental Health Care Act (MHCA), No. 17 of 2002, which replaced the Mental Health Act of 1973, expunged the vestiges of discriminatory legislation on account of the political changes which took place in the country.

Furthermore, the amendments to the South African Criminal Procedure Act have aligned the country with global trends such as a rights-based approach to persons with mental disorders, and respect for fundamental human rights as espoused by international conventions such as the United Nations CRPD.[20]

The implementation of the MHCA has been fraught with challenges such as insufficient human resources as well as funding gaps, but has been quite successful in shifting the emphasis of care from psychiatric facilities to general hospitals, as well as integration into primary care.[21]

Uganda

Uganda's Mental Health Act was passed in 1964, thus replacing the Mental Treatment Act of 1938. The currently existing law does not include safeguards against human rights abuses, and it does not regulate involuntary admission and treatment, seclusion and restraints, special treatments or ethical issues pertaining to research. It still utilizes derogatory and stigmatizing language for persons with mental disorders, such as "idiot", "lunatic" and "imbecile".[22] A revised Mental Treatment Act has been prepared and has been under consideration by the parliament since 2011, and it is expected that when it is eventually ratified, it will bring the country's mental health legislation in line with current rights-based guidelines and best practices.[20]

Conclusion

The road to legislative reform and the passage of updated mental health legislation in SSA is a long and tortuous path, which requires a strong collaborative network of all stakeholders in order to succeed. A sustained advocacy campaign that promotes public awareness, engages the media, service user organizations, non-governmental organizations as well as professional bodies is crucial for the success of this endeavour. Success stories thus far in Ghana and South Africa have required several years of careful planning and sustained advocacy for the end product to be eventually brought to fruition. It is to be hoped that the ripple effects will eventually spread across other SSA countries. This will be a critical first step, ahead of worries about implementation challenges. But what is not in doubt is that effective and updated mental health legislation is a sine qua non for improved mental health services and the protection of the rights of persons with mental disorders in SSA.

References

1   Daar AS, Jacobs M, Wall S, Groenewald J, Eaton J, Patel V, dos Santos P, Kagee A, Gevers A, Sunkel C, Andrews G, Daniels I, Ndetei D. (2014). Declaration on mental health in Africa: moving to implementation. 13; 7: 24589. doi: 10.3402/gha.v7.24589.

2   World Health Organization. (2005). WHO resource book on mental health, human rights and legislation. Geneva: World Health Organization.

3   United Nations. (1948). Universal Declaration of Human Rights. Geneva: United Nations.

4   United Nations. (1991). Principles for the protection of persons with mental illness and the improvement of mental health care. New York: United Nations, Secretariat Centre for Human Rights.

5.   Council of Europe. (1950). European Convention on Human Rights (Convention for the protection of human rights and fundamental freedoms). Strasbourg: Council of Europe.

6   Organisation of African Unity. (1986). African Charter on Human and Peoples Rights.

7   Kelly BD. (2011). Mental health legislation and human rights in England, Wales and the Republic of Ireland. *International Journal of Law and Psychiatry*, 34(6), 439–454. http://doi.org/10.1016/j.ijlp. 2011.10

.009

8   World Health Organization. (2014). *World Mental Health Atlas*. Geneva: World Health Organization.

9   Morakinyo VO. (1977). The Law and psychiatry in Africa. *African Journal of Psychiatry*, 3, 91-98.

10   Ogunlesi AO, Ogunwale A. (2012). Mental health legislation in Nigeria: current leanings and future yearnings. *International Psychiatry*, 9(3), 62–64.

11   Mental Health Act (2012). Parliament of the Republic of Ghana. Accra.

12   Osei A, Roberts M, Crabbe J. (2011). The new Ghana Mental Health Bill. *International Psychiatry*, 8(1): 8–9.

13   Walker G, Osei A (2017). Mental health law in Ghana. *BJPsych International*, 14(2): 38-39

14. Doku V, Wusu-Takyi A, Awakame J. (2012). Implementing the Mental Health Act in Ghana: any challenges ahead? *Ghana Medical Journal*, 46, 241.

15   Walker G. (2015) Ghana Mental Health Act 846 2012: a qualitative study of the challenges and priorities for implementation. *Ghana Medical Journal*, 49, 266–274.

16   Laws of Nigeria. Lunacy Ordinance, Vol. IV, Cap. 121 (1948). Government Printer.

17   Ogunlesi AO, Ogunwale A, Wet PD, Roos L, Kaliski S. (2012). Forensic psychiatry in Africa: prospects and challenges. *African Journal of Psychiatry*, 15, 3–7.

18   US Government Printing Office. (1949). Tribunals of war criminals before the Nuremberg Military Tribunals under Control Council Law No. 10. Washington D.C: US Government Printing Office.

19   World Medical Association. (1949). WMA International Code of Medical Ethics. London: World Medical Association.

20   Mugisha J, Abdulmalik J, Hanlon C, Petersen I, Lund C, Upadhaya N, Ahuja S, Shidhaye R, Mntambo N, Alem A, Gureje O, Kigozi F. (2017). Health systems context(s) for integrating mental health into primary health care in six Emerald countries: a situation analysis. *International Journal of Mental Health Systems* 11:7. doi: 10.1186/s13033-016-0114-2.

21   Ramlall S. (2012). The Mental Health Care Act No 17 -South Africa. Trials and triumphs: 2002-2012. *Afr J Psychiatry*. 15(6):407-10.

22. Cooper S, Ssebunnya J, Kigozi F, Lund C, Flisher A; The Mhapp Research Programme Consortium. (2010). Viewing Uganda's mental health system through a human rights lens. *International Review of Psychiatry*. 22(6):578-88. doi: 10.3109/09540261.2010.536151.

Learning points & objectives

- Mental health legislation is essential for the provision of a legal framework that protects and promotes the rights of persons with mental disorders.

- Only 55% of SSA countries have stand-alone mental health legislation with majority of these laws being obsolete and containing derogatory and stigmatizing language, which are in conflict with current best practices.

- A human rights-based approach is currently recommended for mental health legislation, which should be in tandem with international conventions such as the United Nations' Convention on the Rights of Persons with Disabilities (CRPD).

- Ghana and South Africa are currently the bright spots in terms of the quality of their mental health legislation in SSA; while Nigeria, Uganda and some other countries are pushing for the legislative consideration of their Mental Health Draft Bills.

- The journey to successful passage of contemporary mental health legislation requires patient and persistent advocacy as well as engagement of all stakeholders.

INDEX

245

health care expansion in SSA
  barriers to the provision of, 5
  lack of data for meaningful
    planning, 9
HIV-related dementia, 175
  causative factors, 176
  prevalence in SSA, 176-177

illness and culture in SSA, 20
  symptom severity, 21, 24
  seeking health care in SSA,
    22
  religious and native doctors,
    22
  and Christian faith healers,
    23
  traditional healers tech-
    niques, 23-24
  divination & incantations,
    24
  the social network, 24-25
  need for a complementary
    approach, 31-32
intellectual disability
  defined, 123
  world wide prevalence, 123
  in low and middle income
    countries, 124
  deficits in adaptive func-
    tioning, 126
  causes in enfants and young
    children, 127-128
  and the environment, 128
  nomenclature, 128
  difficulties in diagnosing
    other mental health
    issues, 130
  common health conditions
    associated with, 131
  factors which contribute to

other health issues and
  socialization, 132-133
assessing an ID person for
  other health issues, 133-
  134
treatment options, 135-136
health care delivery, multi-
  disciplinary team, 140
life expectancy, 136
in the undergraduate medical curriculum, 136-138
educational provision for ID
  people, 138
  inclusive or exclusive, 139
  barriers to education, 139
  in Nigeria, 139, 146
  shortage of teachers for
    special needs child-
    ren,139
  in the community, 141-
    142
  and the juvenile justice
    system, 142
  special school in south-
    western Nigeria, 147
legal rights, 142-145
in sub-Saharan Africa, 146

Kenya
  and per capita expenditure
    on mental health, 172

Lambo, Thomas
  colonial rule and mental
    health treatment in
    Nigeria, 41
  developed a community-
    based mental health
    centre in Aro, Abeokuta,
    47

Printed in the United States
By Bookmasters